In his third book, Dr Kanji draws directly on his own research and a wide literature to make sophisticated research both engaging and accessible. He stimulates us to see the connections between common mental health problems, and gives impetus to age-old solutions like exercise, sleep, slow breathing and meditation. And in so doing helps to put us back in control.

John A. Windsor FRSNZ
Professor of Surgery, University of Auckland

This book is a journey of discovery fuelled by Dr Kanji's own health struggles. The connection between stress and insomnia, anxiety and depression has been thoroughly researched in this book. As we are all different, the variety of methods for helping us deal with our stress related health problems are useful and all supported by sound scientific evidence. A great read that makes us think about what we are doing each day and how we can improve our quality of life.

Associate Professor Rachel Page
School of Health Sciences, Massey University

AF583334

Nothing is more powerful than a patient perspective. I like the way Dr Giresh Kanji weaves his personal experience with well researched evidence which makes this book a compelling read. Dr Kanji's passion and lifelong commitment to make connections between the science of stress and his personal experiences makes this book a rare find in its category. An amazing and stimulating book elegantly demystifying a complex jigsaw puzzle.

Professor (Adj) Anil Thapliyal
Centre for eHealth, Faculty of Health and Environmental Sciences, Auckland University of Technology

An astonishing book for the problems of our time. Dr Kanji explains the science with evidence uncovering new information and novel solutions. This book is a must read for both laypeople and health professionals.

Professor Bruce Arroll
University of Auckland

This book is dedicated to all those who suffer from mental illness or have lost loved ones to mental illness.

BRAIN CONNECTIONS

HOW TO SLEEP BETTER, WORRY LESS AND FEEL HAPPIER

DR GIRESH KANJI

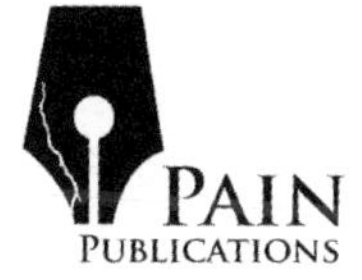

First published in 2019 by Pain Publications,
78 Lambton Quay, Wellington, New Zealand

Copyright © Giresh Kanji 2019

No part of this publication may be stored or transmitted in any form or by any means, electronic or mechanical including recording or storage of any information in a retrieval system, without permission in writing from the publisher.

No reproduction may be made, whether by photocopying or any other means, unless a written licence has been obtained from the author.

National Library of New Zealand Cataloguing-in-Publication Data
Kanji, Giresh, 1966-
Brain Connections: How to Sleep Better, Worry Less and Feel Happier
Author; Giresh Kanji
Includes bibliographical references.
ISBN 978-0-473-46743-2

Cover Design Luke Williamson

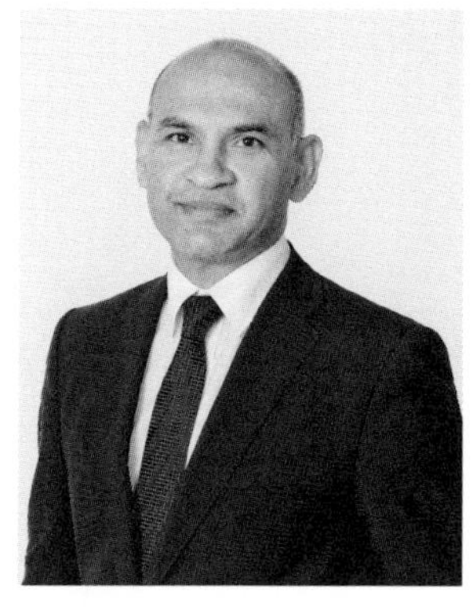

Dr Giresh Kanji was born in Wellington, New Zealand, and educated at Wellington College, Otago Medical School and Massey University. He finished a PhD investigating chronic pain in 2013. He has worked as a medical doctor since 1990 and has been studying at university for over 25 years. After completion of his studies, he founded the New Zealand Pain Foundation to carry out research into chronic pain and mental health disorders. He is currently supervising research on back pain and depression. In 2014 he was appointed the editor of the Australasian Musculoskeletal Medicine Journal. He is an honorary senior lecturer at Auckland University. This book is Dr Kanji's third book and follows "Fix Your Back" and "Fix Your Neck Pain, Headache and Migraine". Giresh is married with three children.

CONTENTS

FOREWORD

Dr Giresh Kanji has long been a passionate advocate for a more holistic approach to health. In this, his third book, he draws on more than two decades of research, clinical practice and his own personal health struggles, to shed light on the causes and potential cures for one of the epidemics of our time: poor sleep, anxiety and depression.

He has an all-too-rare ability to communicate complex scientific concepts simply and succinctly. But you shouldn't mistake simplicity and succinctness for being superficial: his approach is firmly grounded in an in-depth grasp of the extensive scientific evidence on the way stress can harm our health and of the simple, affordable and practical steps we can take to deal with it.

I like the way he doesn't promise magic bullets or promote quick fixes. Instead, Dr Kanji's philosophy is a more credible and pragmatic one: try this evidence-based approach; if that option isn't helping, consider another from the diverse menu he discusses, from meditation through to medication.

In our fast-paced world we all need to take better care of ourselves. This book goes a long way to explaining why and how we can do this. It has helped me to take steps to reduce the adverse effects of stress on my own health. I hope you find this book as informative and instructive to read as I have.

Dr Chris Bullen
Professor of Public Health, University of Auckland

INTRODUCTION

Everyone deserves to live a life free of insomnia, anxiety and depression. The truth is that these symptoms haunt many of us. We have no idea of why they occur and what habits will eliminate these symptoms to let us live a life full of energy and joy. Once symptoms develop they may continue for years and decades, and have a devastating effect on our wellbeing and ability to function at our best. The statistics are sobering: people with major depression have up to 27 times the completed suicide rate compared to people without depression. With medications unable to make a significant impact on some people's lives, new paradigms need to be explored.

Since leaving college in 1986, and working for many years as a doctor, I have enrolled at university or studied for professional papers nearly every year until 2013 when I finished my PhD — a total of 27 years. My thesis examined how stress increases pain, and in this process I discovered how stress creates the symptoms of insomnia, anxiety and depression. My biggest lesson was to keep asking "why" until a logical answer is found. As well as being able to help my patients, my journey has enabled me to break free of the shackles of my own post-traumatic stress disorder. For more than three decades, I was plagued by poor sleep, irritability, night sweats and regular nightmares.

I start with my personal journey in this book. I hope this book offers people suffering stress-related illnesses an explanation of their symptoms, and treatment options that go beyond medications, leading to a long-term cure, and a happier life.

CHAPTER 1

MY STORY – 35 YEARS OF NIGHTMARES

I lay in bed mid-morning, unshaven and unwashed. I felt like the weight of the world was crushing me. I dreaded getting out of bed to face the world and just wanted to hide under the sheets. Usually I woke at the crack of dawn, but now I felt there was little to live for. I turned over and buried my face in the pillow, trying to forget the world outside the four walls of my bedroom.

It had been weeks since I last left the house. I had lost interest in running, swimming, playing hockey or even eating. I couldn't recall the last time I shaved or had a shower. I don't know why I felt this way. I was the opposite of happy, depressed and no fun to be around. Even my girlfriend had ended our relationship, noticing the changes over the past month.

It was the summer of 1986, and I was 20, depressed and alone. I felt embarrassed. It was the summer holidays and I was home from studying medicine in Dunedin. What did I have to be depressed about? I was realising my childhood dream of becoming a doctor, a dream I had held since I was seven years old. I recall going to the dental clinic with my mother. The receptionist asked,

"What are you going to do when you grow up?" I said, "I am going to be a doctor."

My mother knocked on the door and shouted my name. She had tried to get me out of bed for the past week. I just told her I had the flu. One day I woke up, decided to put on my running gear and went for a run. After that first run, I took a shower and felt refreshed for the first time in a month. I even took off the beard. I had run regularly since the age of 12 and had forgotten how good it felt. The next day, and the next day, I just put on my running shoes and ran around the hills of Wellington. After a few weeks my bed no longer was my safe place. I started seeing friends, my appetite had returned, and I was returning to a happier place. Fortunately, classes did not start for six weeks. I slowly developed enough social and mental resilience to return to university. After this episode, my self-esteem took a nosedive with a loss of confidence that took over six months to return.

My experience of hospitals started well before my medical school days. In 1970, at the age of four, I was diagnosed with tuberculosis and spent three months in isolation at the fever hospital in Mt Victoria. I remember spending a lot of time in a dark room with few windows. I suspect I had an injection every day, but cannot remember this time with much clarity.

My mother came to visit every day, bringing me food and love. That was probably the only thing that kept me going, knowing she would come back the next day. Every two weeks we would see the specialist, who told my mother and me that I could leave in two weeks. I was so happy to hear this, but every time we had our next meeting he said the same thing. Two weeks stretched out to three long months before I finally went home.

A year later my family were driving down Tasman St, Wellington. It was very exciting as we were going to the movies with Dad. It was a wet April day and to this day I do not know exactly what went wrong but the truck we were sitting in swerved onto the other side of the road. Boom – a large car went straight into the side of our truck. The next thing I knew was waking up in the emergency department of Wellington Hospital. It was frightening, all my six brothers and sisters going in different directions to be checked for their injuries. Luckily no one died and all my brothers and sisters developed only minor bruising. I was in incredible agony and passed out. I had fractured my hip.

The memories from this hospital admission are more vivid. My leg was in traction for over two months as I lay there watching the world pass me by. The first night was special as my little brother was admitted into hospital for observation and crept into my bed and spent the night with me. I remember the school teacher; her very kind face is still etched in my memory bank. She would come with her trolley full of books. I don't recall reading any books but remember her kind manner as if I were lying in that hospital bed today.

Being a child in a hospital bed you get a bit spoiled. The nurses would cut up my poached eggs on toast for breakfast. The thing I remember the most was my brothers and sisters visiting. We would play cards and talk about what we were going to do once I left the hospital – go for picnics, travel and play cricket and rugby. The memory of them leaving is still vivid in my mind. My tears would well up and I would cry myself to sleep once they had left.

One Sunday I remember them telling me to look out of the window. There it was, a new car that we could squeeze the whole family into – a Holden Kingswood with six seats and four doors, a significant upgrade from the Thames 500 truck with two doors and two seats. The second-hand car was a source of joy for many years as we travelled the length of New Zealand to visit friends and see the country.

Once I left hospital I returned to Berhampore School. I integrated back into school but always felt a little anxious. Sometimes about what I wore, sometimes about whether I fitted in and sometimes about whether I was liked by others. I was also very irritable and certainly not relaxed. Worst of all I would wake with nightmares and night sweats on a regular basis, often several times a week. The most recurrent nightmare was walking down Cuba St with my family. It was dark and just as we walk past a busker, playing a guitar in a bowler hat, he lifts me up and runs off with me into the dark. All I can hear is the screaming of my mother as I wake up drenched in sweat with my heart pounding.

I would frequently have other nightmares: about failing exams, about being chased or being delayed when going to a crucial engagement. Sometimes I could not open a door that was inexplicably stuck, sometimes I would miss a bus and sometimes I would be just plain lost, not having a clue what street I was on. The things I would miss most often were exams and flights. The nightmares continued until I was 40 years old.

In my last year of medical school my fortunes took a turn for the better. I fell in love and somebody actually fell in love with me. Not only was she beautiful, but she was always smiling, happy and laughing — a real joy to be around. Her sense of fun was matched by her dependability, helping to bring some stability and calm into my life. I married her at the age of 25, and for over 25 years she has been there for me.

My wife navigated me through the rough water that was my life. Sleep disturbances were often accompanied by a foul temper and irritability, interspersed with some calm patches. The night sweats were so frequent that my sheets and pillowcase would discolour and become a shade of yellow. Over time, as I thrashed my legs, the sheets would develop holes, needing frequent replacement. Looking back, many women would have run for the hills rather than deal with me and my moods.

We had three children in the space of five years. I remember when my first was born, the first six months were like a hurricane where you do not get the chance to catch your breath. We never knew what to expect. We were lucky that both our parents lived in the city, not far away. My in-laws were always available to help us get through this testing time that was also filled with the joy of bringing someone new into the world. A patient once said to me "the most exciting time in your life is watching your children grow up" and looking back I can say he was right.

Three young children provided plenty of challenges to both of us. I somehow knew that I could not work too hard, otherwise I may not cope. Some inbuilt protection mechanism kicked in that ensured I had time to look after myself and my young family.

I spent most of my 20s, 30s and 40s enrolled at university doing various degrees and diplomas. I really enjoyed learning, and becoming a critical thinker has helped me make sense of my life, and hopefully can help others as well.

I enrolled in a PhD to focus on how pain spreads and amplifies. I investigated the relationship between pain, mood and sleep. I would wake at 5 am and read medical papers until I literally fell asleep on the couch watching television in the evenings. I read thousands of medical papers and made thousands of internet searches during this time. I spent five years doing this, trying to make connections between the science of stress and my personal experiences.

The reading on pain, mood, sleep and heat started making sense of my world and the world around me. My suspicion was gaining momentum – the sympathetic nervous system (stress nervous system) activates both pain and stress related conditions. Treatment aimed at reducing stress nervous system activity would be a powerful ally against these conditions.

I started to form a hypothesis: that heat was likely to be a weapon in reducing the activity of the stress nervous system. I refocused my searches into the effects of heat on the stress pathways of the body, opening a whole new body of knowledge I was previously unaware of. I even started attending the sauna and hot yoga regularly, and noted benefits for my own stress related symptoms.

The next chapter discusses the inner workings of the stress nervous system, to explore how stress operates in every facet of our lives.

CHAPTER 2

BRAIN CONNECTIONS – THE INNER WORKINGS OF THE BRAIN

Electrical impulses in our brain ultimately control the sensations we are experiencing. The level of electricity in different parts of our brain can shape many phenomena, including migraine, epilepsy, insomnia, anxiety and depression. Things that happen to us and our reaction to them based on previous experiences shape how the electrical circuits in the brain behave. Let's look at migraine and epilepsy first.

A migraine aura occurs when someone experiences a visual experience usually in the form of a blurred image. Sometimes a migraine aura can be an odour. They experience a smell when nothing is in front of them. The sensation originates in the brain due to spontaneous sparks of electricity. If a person experiences a visual aura, then a spark of electricity is generated in the visual part of the brain. If a person experiences an odour, then the part of the brain responsible for smell is sparking electricity.

Classic epilepsy occurs when a spark of electricity flashes within the part of the brain concerned with movement (motor cortex). Hence a person with epilepsy starts to shake rhythmically. The migraine aura and the epileptic seizure are basically the same phenomena occurring in different parts of the human brain. The medications used to reduce attacks of migraine and epilepsy aim to reduce the electricity in the brain to reduce the occurrence of episodes.

People with migraine and epilepsy have electrical channels in the brain that open up quicker, so they produce more electricity in certain parts of the brain. The level of electricity produced corresponds to the severity of symptoms experienced. To understand the severity of symptoms experienced by people with migraine, we can look at electricity transmission.

In those without migraine, if five microvolts of electricity are produced by the body, five microvolts may arrive at the brain. However, with migraine, five microvolts may increase to 50 microvolts in the part of the brain involved with sensations (sensory cortex), increasing the severity of sensory symptoms such as light, sound, touch, smell and pain. Accordingly, during a migraine attack, people prefer to lie in a dark, quiet room. People with migraine experience more pain (low back pain, headache pain, neck pain and fibromyalgia) than people who do not experience migraine.

Symptoms of migraine aura and epilepsy are due to electrical activity in different parts of the brain. I started exploring the notion that other symptoms, such as insomnia, anxiety and depression, could also be caused by electrical activity in the brain: specifically, activity in the reticular formation for insomnia and in the amygdala for anxiety and panic attacks.

In depression, symptoms can be explained by changes in electrical activity in parts of the brain, including the reticular formation, amygdala and the hypothalamus. Electricity is increased in some parts and decreased in others; this can occur when receptors are repeatedly hit over time by stress chemicals.

People with migraine and epilepsy do not have symptoms all the time. They are often perfectly well in between episodes. The same is often true for the symptoms of insomnia, anxiety and depression. The real question is: "what causes the flashes of electricity that give rise to symptoms of migraine, epilepsy, insomnia, anxiety and depression?" The answer may lead to treatments that can switch off the electricity and help patients with these symptoms.

I wanted to explore whether the human stress response was the likely reason for increased electrical discharges in the brain, leading to migraine attacks and stress related symptoms.

CHAPTER 3

HOW DOES YOUR BODY RESPOND TO STRESS?

Professor Walter Cannon, from Harvard Medical School, first described the stress response, or "fight or flight" response as it is better known, in 1915. When a human being is under threat, the brain orchestrates the release of neurotransmitters and hormones throughout the brain and body to prepare us for intense physical activity, such as running or fighting.

The stress response activates all the senses, including sight, sound, touch and smell, and keeps us alert and anxious by activating electricity in nearly every part of the brain. At least six stress chemicals are released in the brain, including adrenaline, noradrenaline, serotonin, histamine, corticotrophin-releasing hormone and acetylcholine. The stress response also prepares the whole body to fight or flee, by releasing adrenaline, noradrenaline and cortisol from the adrenal gland into the bloodstream.

A coordinated change in blood flow occurs throughout the body. Blood flow is drawn away from non-essential organs such as the gut, kidney, liver and immune system, and diverted to muscles involved in running and fighting. Blood flow to the muscles can increase ten-fold, while blood flow is reduced to the hands and feet. This is the reason why cold hands and feet are a symptom of an overactive stress nervous system.

The heart contracts faster and more vigorously to increase blood flow to the muscles. Many people experience a thumping awareness of their heartbeat called palpitations. Blood vessels also constrict throughout the body, increasing blood pressure. Fuel in the form of glucose and fats is released into the blood stream. The high blood pressure and increased glucose and fats in the blood stream are the reasons why stress is a major risk factor for heart attacks.

Blood flow to the abdominal organs can reduce as much as 40 percent, since digestion is less important than immediate survival. Gastric secretions can also reduce as much as 40 percent, contributing to irritable bowel syndrome.

When stress chemicals are released in the brain, they attach to receptors and create electrical discharges. The part of a person's brain where electrical discharges are most active will determine their immediate symptoms. Staying awake (insomnia) and being anxious were crucial to survival when faced with danger. They are an immediate response of the brain that has been flooded with stress chemicals. Depression often develops later.

There is significant overlap for insomnia, anxiety

and depression, since all three symptoms are exacerbated by the stress response. Patients rarely have only one of these three symptoms. In a large population study looking at insomnia, the authors found 75 percent of those with poor sleep suffered from a mood disorder such as depression, and 64 percent suffered from anxiety.[1]

CHAPTER 4

WINDING UP THE STRESS NERVOUS SYSTEM

If the stress nervous system is activated repeatedly it winds up to become exquisitely sensitive. Psychological stress, illness, viral infection, chronic pain, nightmares, smoking, alcohol and intense concentration all activate the stress response. However, if the stress chemicals released are not depleted by running or fighting, they flood the brain and body. Neurons in the brain can become sensitive and stress organs in the brain and body can enlarge.

Messages transmitted by nerves are subject to change, and their strength can be altered by several mechanisms. When one nerve connects to another nerve, at a junction called the synapse, it releases chemicals that attach to the next nerve to continue the message. The amount of chemicals released at the synapse can either amplify or weaken the signal. Normally only 30 percent of chemicals bind to the second nerve; however, this can increase to 80 percent to increase the strength of the message. New synapses can also grow, sensitising the nervous system.

A study performed on medical students 40 years ago illustrates the powerful enhancing effect of winding up messages in the brain.[2] Students were exposed to light from a torch, then given a drug called scoline that causes paralysis for one minute. The students reacted to the paralysis with extreme panic as you would expect as students could not breathe when paralysed. Afterwards, whenever the students were exposed to the light, the same panic reaction was seen without injecting scoline, despite there being no rational connection between the light and the paralysis.

The parts of the brain and body producing stress chemicals, such as the pituitary gland and adrenal gland, grow. The pathways also become more efficient. So if two people experience exactly the same stress, the person with the wound up stress nervous system releases more stress chemicals. Once the stress nervous system winds up, it can remain wound up for life, predisposing an individual to a lifetime of stress related illnesses.

The activity of the stress nervous system is measured using heart rate variability. Several studies have compared heart rate variability for people with and without stress related illness. Studies have found the activity of the stress nervous system is elevated in insomnia,[3] panic attacks, obsessive–compulsive, generalised, and social anxiety disorders,[4] depression,[5] bipolar disorder and schizophrenia.[6] When this phenomenon was studied for depression at Ruhr-University of Bochum in Germany, they found the degree of depression correlates positively with the level of activity of the stress nervous system.[7] The same researchers also found a reduction in activity of the stress nervous system with successful treatment of depression.[8]

Smoking, alcohol and concentration also activate the stress response. The Department of Cardiology, Kosuyolu Research Hospital, Istanbul, Turkey investigated the effect of smoking on the stress nervous system.[9] Smoking was shown to increase the activity of the stress nervous system, and therefore is likely to exacerbate stress related symptoms including insomnia, anxiety and depression. Researchers at Boston University School of Medicine, in the United States, found increased stress nervous system activity in depressed patients who smoked compared with those who did not.[10] Smoking is likely to reduce the likelihood of recovery from insomnia, anxiety or depression.

Alcohol in small quantities relaxes a person; however, more than a few glasses increases stress chemicals and disturbs sleep. Several studies have shown alcohol increases the activity of the stress nervous system.[11,12,13] One of these studies found that one 150ml glass of wine did not elevate the activity of the stress nervous system but two glasses (300ml) did. The hangover headache that develops overnight after binge drinking is likely to be due to the gradual build up of stress chemicals increasing electricity in the pain centres of the brain.

Alcohol can also trigger headache and migraine with one or two glasses through the same mechanism.

Concentration increases stress chemicals, and if someone has a wound up stress nervous system, this can cause symptoms. Increased concentration around deadlines such as exams, or delivering work projects, will lead to increased activity of the stress nervous system and aggravate insomnia, anxiety and depression.

Our current sedentary lifestyle is at odds with our bodies, which have developed over millions of years to serve humans who have been hunters, gatherers and predators. Activation of the stress pathways in human beings, without depletion of stress chemicals, is leading to an alarming increase in stress related illnesses.

CHAPTER 5

THE ROLE OF CHILDHOOD TRAUMA

The research is clear when it comes to childhood trauma. People with childhood trauma experience more stress related symptoms as their stress nervous systems have wound up and become more sensitive to life stressors. Several studies show children who suffer ongoing or repeated trauma, such as psychological abuse, physical abuse, parental loss and other adverse conditions, are at increased risk of experiencing insomnia, anxiety, panic attacks and depression.[14,15,16]

Researchers at Harvard University, in the United States, showed that children who were maltreated were 300 percent more likely to experience mood disorders and 200 percent more likely to experience anxiety.[14] A study by the Department of Psychiatry and Human Genetics, Commonwealth University, Virginia, in the United States, found that 2,000 females who had experienced parent separation before the age of 17 were at increased risk of anxiety, depression and panic disorder.[15]

The department of Preventive Medicine, Southern California Permanente Medical Group in San Diego studied the link between childhood trauma and stress related symptoms.[17] They mailed out a questionnaire about adverse childhood experiences to 13,494 adults with around 7,500 respondents and found childhood trauma predisposed to poor health. The study looked at exposure to physical, psychological and sexual abuse, alcoholism, drug abuse and mental illness within the family.

Approximately 50 percent of people reported at least one type of significant childhood trauma. Six percent experienced more than four different types of childhood trauma when growing up. As children were exposed to more stresses, they were more likely to develop depression and attempt suicide as an adult.

Children exposed to one stressor were twice as likely to have depression and attempt suicide. Children exposed to four or more stressors were five times more likely to become depressed and 12 times more likely to attempt suicide. Similar findings were found for alcoholism and drug abuse. People exposed to one stressor were twice as likely to consider themselves alcoholics, and if four or more stressors were present people were seven times more likely to consider themselves alcoholics. People with one risk factor were twice as likely to use illicit drugs and those with four or more risk factors were five times more likely to use illicit drugs.

In Japan nearly 1,600 Japanese university students

hospitalised from a stress related illness were studied to examine their life experiences.[18] The reason this became important to study was a disturbing trend. During the 1990s there was an increase in the number of children admitted to hospital with stress related illness such as irritable bowel syndrome, headache, depression, hyperventilation syndrome and eating disorders. This was perceived as due to stress arising from academic competition, poor relationships with classmates or teachers in schools and poor parental interaction.

This study looked at factors that may increase a person's risk of developing stress related illness and looked at an individual's interaction with their family and life outside the family. They documented family factors including witnessing domestic violence, physical violence, emotional abuse, illness in the household, parental separation or divorce, little affection from parents and a dysfunctional family. They also documented what was going on outside the family including physical violence, negative recognition by teachers, being bullied in elementary or junior high school and sexual violence.

Of the 1,600 people interviewed 600 people experienced stressful factors within the family and more than 700 experienced stressful factors away from home. The study found adverse childhood experiences, such as emotional abuse and an illness in the household, almost doubled the person's chance of stress related illness. The experience of being bullied in school or physical violence by teachers or classmates increased the person's risk of stress related illness by 250 percent. The more factors a person experienced the higher their risk of stress related illness became.

Childhood trauma is not needed to wind up the stress nervous system. The stress nervous system can wind up before you are born in your mother's womb. Two studies performed by the University of Miami Medical School (in collaboration with other researchers) have found levels of stress chemicals such as adrenaline, noradrenaline and cortisol are elevated in depressed pregnant mothers.[19,20] Babies born to depressed mothers also had elevated levels of stress chemicals in their bloodstream and greater activity of the stress nervous system. Any significant and prolonged stress during pregnancy is likely to raise the levels of stress chemicals in the baby while in the womb. Once sensitivity has increased and the stress nervous system is wound up, everyday small stressors release more stress chemicals in babies, which can carry on for many years and decades leading to stress related symptoms.

Our early life experiences are critical in shaping our lives. Our ability to cope with the future is compromised and the downward spiral of poor mental health can lead to a life without joy. Once our stress nervous system has been wound up, it plagues us for decades. It has been found that once you develop depression, it is easier for further episodes of depression to develop because your stress nervous system winds up further with each episode. Insomnia and anxiety are likely to follow the same pattern.

I recently met Vivian who was born during the Second World War in London. During the war things were turned upside down. Getting to sleep seemed impossible. There was the fear of bombings and the noise of the warning sirens as well as just being in a difficult place. She told me she rarely slept and most nights just placed her head under the sheets and lay awake.

If the war was not enough to contend with her parents were also divorced, and she lived with her mother in financially difficult times. Even at the very young age of seven, she recalls wondering why she was alive and how long she would have to endure living. There was no joy in her world. To make matters worse her mother could no longer look after her and she was sent to live with her father and stepmother. She had little to do with her father or stepmother prior to this and it was like going to live with complete strangers. At the age of 12, she felt every day was a chore rather than the beginning of a new day. On many occasions she thought how nice it would be to go to sleep and never wake up.

Vivian had disturbed sleep for most of her life. She would get to sleep easily but would often wake at 1.30

am and take an hour to get back to sleep. She also felt tired and from her tragic start was robbed of the joy for living. Mostly she hoped her life would not go on for too long. When I met her she was 83 years old. Her mood had improved and she was happier now than she had ever been. She had started meditating many years ago and felt this helped her cope.

I have discussed the wound up stress nervous system. Another critical event occurs in the human brain with repeated stress that helps explain why insomnia, anxiety and depression are recurrent disorders rather than one off problems. As I explained previously, electricity in the brain is the precursor to many symptoms we experience. On one side we have the stress response increasing electricity in many parts of the brain. Normally there are pathways in the brain that suppress electricity, acting like an off switch. These brain neurones act on GABA, a neurotransmitter that shuts off electrical channels. Sleeping tablets like Valium (diazepam) act on GABA receptors to reduce electricity in the brain and help people sleep. Approximately 20 percent of all neurones in the brain produce GABA.[21] Suppression of electricity throughout the brain is a very important phenomenon.

Prolonged stress reduces GABA levels throughout the brain. Researchers at Harvard University compared groups of people with and without insomnia, finding people with insomnia had a 30 percent reduction in brain GABA levels.[22] Researchers at Yale University found GABA was 22 percent lower in a group of people with panic disorder when compared to a group without panic disorder.[23]

The same researchers at Yale compared the levels of GABA in a group of depressed individuals and a group of individuals without depression, finding a 52 percent reduction in GABA levels in people experiencing depression.[24] Both the stress response and the loss of GABA are likely to perpetuate stress related symptoms of insomnia, anxiety and depression.

Insomnia, anxiety and depression are symptoms. Unlike infections such as pneumonia where a cause is present, symptoms have no apparent cause or cure in modern medicine but are managed for the patient's entire life at a significant medical and personal cost. The costs of medical reviews, pharmaceuticals, alternative therapies and vitamins escalate quickly.

These unexplained symptoms are ruining millions of lives around the world. The medical profession has not been able to explain these symptoms enough to advise people of a logical explanation that leads to logical solutions. Instead, a trial and error approach has to be used. The cause of symptoms needs to be targeted to obtain a cure. Medications can often help short term but often work poorly long term for insomnia, anxiety and depression. As doctors we will prescribe one medication to target the end of the chain, rather than explain the development of symptoms and lifelong solutions to their problems.

One useful analogy is the historical discovery of infectious agents such as pneumonia. Before the causes of infectious diseases were discovered, doctors were forced to treat patients with a hit and miss approach. It was only after infectious agents were identified that a logical approach could be used to find treatments such as antibiotics, vaccines, and antivirals.

What I aim to present in this book is the evidence that leads to a coherent explanation of symptoms. Therefore I aim to identify treatments for the cause of patients' symptoms. Once patients understand their symptoms they are much more likely to create the habits that will improve their symptoms in the long term.

CHAPTER 6

WHAT IS SLEEP?

Sleep is the barometer of mental, spiritual and physical wellbeing. Waking feeling invigorated and refreshed is one of life's great joys. Having energy, joyfulness and a spark for life are all linked to a good night's sleep. Scientists struggle to answer the question of why we sleep. However, scientists all agree that poor sleep has an adverse effect on nearly every aspect of our health. The most important function of sleep is to reduce the activity of the stress nervous system. Poor sleep leads to an over-active stress nervous system, compromising our health and resilience to what happens to us on a day to day basis.

Sleep and wakefulness are determined by electrical activity in the brain, particularly in the reticular formation. The reticular formation is a part of the brain that regulates sleep and arousal. If the reticular formation is damaged, then people can fall into a state of deep sleep (coma). Increased electrical activity in the reticular formation causes you to stay awake (insomnia). While we are awake, electricity is increased and while we are asleep electricity is reduced.

So how does stress give rise to insomnia? During

the stress response our stress chemicals bind to receptors in the reticular formation and increase electricity. This causes wakefulness. Some neurotransmitters, such as GABA, can reduce electrical activity in the brain, inducing sleepiness. Sleeping tablets target these receptors in the brain.

Sleep is made up of five phases: one, two, three, four and Rapid Eye Movement (REM) sleep. Stages one and two are light sleep, while stages three and four are deep sleep. We often dream during REM sleep. If we wake in deep sleep, we often feel groggy and if we wake during REM sleep we can sometimes recall our dreams. Rapid Eye Movement sleep takes up around 20 percent of our total sleep time. During REM sleep our eyes jerk in various directions and our legs and arms become paralysed. We cannot even control our body temperature during REM sleep.

Are We Sleeping Less?

As modern society evolves there is more demand on our time due to work and busier lifestyles. There is less time available for exercise, relaxation and sleep. Changes, such as businesses opening 24 hours a day, seven days a week, have resulted in increased shift work and weekend work, leading to a work-life-family imbalance, eroding our support structures and downtime. Recent changes in technology have exacerbated this trend. Increased connectivity has led to increased screen time, including television, laptops, tablets and especially phones. You can now check your texts, emails and the latest news 24/7, whether at the dinner table or in your bed.

I remember when my children were younger I had a hard and fast rule that no child under my care would have a television in their bedroom as I did not want the children holed up in their bedroom 24 hours a day. As they grew up in the technology age, they had laptops with access to the world. My rule on televisions was irrelevant as they could sit with their laptops in their rooms and entertain themselves. Smartphones have taken this one step further. The world is now accessible through a smartphone from anywhere, all the time.

The average hours a person sleeps have reduced over the past century from 8.3 hours to 6.8 hours. Similar trends are being found across the globe. Researchers from the National Public Health Institute in Finland looked at seven questionnaires dating from 1972 to 2005 and found the number of people sleeping the recommended seven to eight hours has reduced and insomnia-related symptoms increased over this period of time.[25]

In the United States the National Centre for Health Statistics found in 1985, two-thirds of the population slept the recommended seven to eight hours.[26] In 2013, the average sleep duration was six hours 31 minutes on work nights with over half sleeping less than seven hours. Alarming trends are seen in teenagers with more than half of 15 to 17-year-old teenagers sleeping less than seven hours on a school night.

As we are sleeping less we are also doing less physical activity. Most household tasks are now automated, and food is available in plentiful supply from the supermarket. I remember growing up in the 1970s where my parents were avid gardeners and my mum would walk everywhere, to work, to school to drop us off and to the supermarket. Now every family has at least one motor vehicle so walking is reduced. The net effect of less physical activity and busier lives is people having less time to sleep and more difficulty sleeping.

CHAPTER 7

WHAT IS POOR SLEEP?

Poor sleep is characterised by difficulties getting to sleep, staying asleep or waking early in the morning with difficulty getting back to sleep. Insomnia is a public health crisis affecting up to one-third of the population, and costing in the realm of US$100 billion a year in the United States alone. The research has shown that people who develop insomnia often have more life stressors present over the past year, such as death of a spouse, divorce, marital separation, spending time in jail, death of a family member and personal injury or illness. The more stressful events a person experiences the more likely they will experience insomnia.

Research has followed people for several decades to see what trends emerged. Researchers at Kings College Institute of Psychiatry in London followed more than 20,000 people from England for 14 years with three separate surveys carried out in 1993, 2000, and 2007.[27] They found insomnia and the consumption of sleeping tablets doubled during this period. The surveys also found if you experienced insomnia, your risk of depression is 11 times greater and if you experienced insomnia with fatigue your risk of developing depression was 16 times higher than for someone who slept well.

Once the stress nervous system becomes wound up, any new stress releases more stress chemicals, making a person more alert and awake. People can become light sleepers with noises such as the clock ticking, refrigerators or air conditioning disturbing sleep. I remember for many years when I was holidaying the first thing I would do in the hotel room was turn the refrigerator off as I knew this would disturb me. The other main noise that would wake me was the noise of the air-conditioning unit. Much to my wife's dismay I would turn off the air-conditioning unit regardless of the temperature. Even signals such as a half-full bladder will wake people who are light sleepers.

The opposite of a light sleeper is a sleeping baby. They sleep through loud noises, talking or the noise of the television. If you sleep poorly you also have an increased risk of anxiety, depression, heart disease, hypertension, cancer, diabetes, gut disorders, obesity and early death. The risk of developing diabetes increases 30 percent while the risk of obesity increases 50 percent.

If all that was not enough, studies have found poor sleep can lead to an early grave. One study, set in the United States, followed people for 20 years looking at insomnia and death rates. People with persistent poor sleep were three times more likely to die earlier than those who slept well.[28] People who required regular sleeping tablets were four times more likely to die early. Imagine presenting to the doctor and asking for the quick fix to insomnia – sleeping tablets. If the doctor told you the truth, here is your script for sleeping tablets, by the way they are addictive, and if you frequently take sleeping tablets, your chance of dying early increases by 400 percent, would you still take this option?

Once I Have Insomnia Will it Go Away?

The current research shows once you develop insomnia it is likely to persist. A study carried out by Keele University in the United Kingdom showed half of the people studied had trouble falling asleep on some nights and 12 percent experienced trouble falling asleep on most nights.[29] Half of all people woke on some nights and one-quarter of them woke every night. Half of all the people surveyed woke some mornings feeling tired and worn out while 20 percent felt this way every morning. Overall, 37 percent of the population were diagnosed with insomnia. The study followed everyone for one year and found 70 percent continued to experience insomnia. For people with insomnia the risk of developing anxiety increased 200 percent after a year while the risk of developing depression increased by 300 percent.

Another study performed by University Laval in Quebec, Canada also found 74 percent of people continued to experience insomnia one year later.[30]

Uppsala University in Sweden performed a repeat survey of people experiencing insomnia and found 50 percent continued to experience severe sleep disturbance 10 years later.[31]

I have experienced this lifelong trend of poor sleep, sometimes having good spells of a few months and then reverting back to sleep disturbance. Although the nightmares and nights sweats had reduced around the age of 40 my sleep would be disturbed from time to time, probably more disturbed than sound. During 2015, I moved from Wellington to Auckland. I commuted to Wellington for work, had less time to attend the sauna and practise yoga. The stress of moving and commuting disturbed my sleep again. I would wake regularly at night in the early hours of the morning with my heart racing and in a cold sweat.

When your stress nervous system is wound up it is sensitive to anything that releases stress chemicals. I particularly noticed this with alcohol. If I had two to three glasses of wine I would wake in the middle of the night with palpitations, night sweats and wakefulness. If I consumed caffeine after midday, I would have trouble getting to sleep. I recall one particular day having three cups of white tea in the afternoon and evening. I forgot white tea has caffeine. Instead of the usual 10 to 15 minutes to fall asleep it took me more than two hours to get to sleep.

At my worst, I was waking every time I entered a dream phase. During dreams, your brain is very active. When entering this phase of sleep, I instantly woke. As you dream several times a night this was very annoying. I thought I had a heart racing condition so I went to the cardiologist and had a Holter monitor fitted, that measures heart rhythm, strapped to my chest for a few days and nights. There was nothing wrong with my heart. My stress nervous system was wound up to the extent that dreams woke me up.

As well as experiencing sleep disturbance, I fell asleep at the drop of a hat during the day. While on the plane at 7 am I would be asleep before the plane took off until the thump of the landing that would wake me up. Even on the bus home from work, I'd fall asleep and occasionally miss my stop. In the evenings, I would be asleep in front of the television as early as 8 pm. It was only from reading research for this book that I found out falling asleep on the bus, plane or in front of the television was a sign of sleep deprivation. It was not something to marvel at, but a rather significant health issue for me.

My energy also took a nosedive. I had always cycled, played hockey and squash, and enjoyed swimming and going to the gym. I now found it a struggle to go to the gym for 15 to 20 minutes. I started regularly hitting the wall every afternoon and evening. I felt like I was flattened by a bulldozer and it was impossible to pick myself up. I'd grab a heat pack, place it around my neck and lie down in bed most days after dinner. This became even more noticeable on a trip overseas with the change in time zones and my energy faded by 3 pm on some days. I had a whole range of blood tests for my liver, kidney, infections and anaemia – all came back negative. I had finally reached the adrenaline burnout that I had seen in so many patients presenting with chronic fatigue syndrome. This is when the adrenal glands no longer produce enough cortisol, a hormone that gives us energy.

My memory was also in burnout mode. It was failing me. In my late 40s I started forgetting names, places and events. Another worrying pattern was forgetting mid-sentence what I was saying. It was as if my train of thought was suddenly derailed, abandoned in the middle of the railway tracks.

I needed to do something, so I started keeping a sleep diary, recording when I went to bed, woke up and what woke me up during the night. I started eliminating some of the things that were disturbing my sleep. I kept the bedroom door closed so the cat would not wake me. I exercised more regularly and started keeping very regular sleep hours. A few hours before going to sleep I would not engage in activities that required concentration. Within months I started to sleep seven to nine hours with no long wakeful periods. Sometimes

I'd wake during the night, but quietly fall asleep again. Before, I would get up during these wakeful periods, often at five in the morning and start reading or writing.

After sleeping well for three months I noticed I no longer fell asleep during the day and I no longer experienced an all-consuming fatigue in the afternoon that hit me like a ton of bricks. My energy levels and memory started improving. I started remembering names of authors, acquaintances and other small details. I was even managing a 40-minute workout at the gym. I had a new lease of life that led me to pick up this book and finish writing it, something I had put off due to my poor sleep, memory, concentration as well as reduced energy and enthusiasm.

CHAPTER 8

SLEEP HYGIENE

Sleep hygiene measures are recommendations based on clinical observations in the 1970s by Dr Hauri. The recommendations are designed to improve sleep by avoiding behaviours that interfere with sleep and promoting behaviours that enhance good sleep.

Sleep hygiene measures include:

- Curtail time in bed – avoid staying in bed for prolonged periods when you cannot sleep.
- Keep regular times getting to sleep and waking.
- Get regular exercise.
- Avoid an uncomfortable environment – excessive loud noises at night, room too hot or cold, bright lights.
- Avoid coffee, alcohol or nicotine.
- Eat a light snack before bedtime.
- Rather than trying to get to sleep, do something else until you feel tired then return to sleep.
- Eliminate the bedroom clock.
- Explore napping/avoid napping.

- Use occasional sleeping tablets, but not regular sleeping tablets as regular use is ineffective.
- Avoid stimulation prior to sleep such as exercise, arguments and activities requiring high levels of concentration.

Insomniacs have poorer sleep hygiene than people who sleep well. People with insomnia are more likely to nap, smoke, sleep in on non-working days and take alcohol.[28] Despite this finding it is hard to distinguish whether these habits are a consequence of poor sleep or whether these habits caused poor sleep. For example, if someone was having a bad patch with their sleep they may be tired and start to have afternoon naps. They may also start to drink alcohol in the false belief this will help them sleep.

The list of sleep hygiene habits is an important check list to ensure the sleep environment is optimal for a good night's sleep. I would recommend going through the list to eliminate barriers to a good night sleep such as noise, temperature, pet disturbances and light. Habits such as keeping a regular sleep time and avoiding stimulating activities prior to sleep will also help reduce sleep disturbance. The next chapter will discuss factors that can disturb sleep.

CHAPTER 9

FACTORS THAT CAN DISTURB SLEEP

The mind and body work as a finely tuned system with the hypothalamus, a centre in the brain, responsible for temperature control, appetite and stress. The hypothalamus keeps the mind-body in balance. If the body becomes too hot, the hypothalamus promotes sweating to reduce body temperature, or if the body becomes too cold, shivering occurs to heat the body up. Anything that upsets this balance increases the activity of the stress nervous system and can disturb sleep.

Temperature and Sleep

Changes in temperature can disturb sleep. We have all experienced this in the middle of winter when temperature plummets or the middle of summer as the mercury surges. Once the body cools or heats, the stress nervous system is activated to heat or cool the body respectively.

Snoring and Sleep Apnoea

Snoring disturbs partners due to the noise and can also disturb an individual's sleep. Snoring is a result of relaxation of muscles that keep the airway open when awake. The flow of air as we breath causes vibration of the airways creating the noise of snoring.

Sleep apnoea is when people stop breathing during the night repeatedly due to obstruction of the breathing passages. Sleep apnoea disturbs an individual's sleep, reduces energy for exercise and can set up a spiral leading to weight gain. This vicious cycle can be very difficult to break. Many devices such as jaw splints and continuous positive airway pressure can help with sleep apnoea.

Alcohol

Many of us know that a glass of wine or a beer can be very relaxing. However, most of us are unaware that more than a few glasses of alcohol can have exactly the opposite effect by increasing the activity of the stress nervous system. More than one glass of wine can disturb sleep by inducing a light sleep and reducing REM sleep. Many people self-medicate by taking alcohol to help them cope with stress and sleep. Unfortunately excess alcohol does exactly the opposite, reducing one's ability to cope with stress and sleep.

Concentration

Concentration activates the stress nervous system and releases stress chemicals. Doing activities that require concentration are best stopped a few hours prior to sleeping to give the brain a chance to unwind. I recall as a young hospital doctor when shifts would end at midnight, it would take several hours to get to sleep as I would feel wound up when getting home.

Smoking

Smoking can keep people awake for two reasons. Firstly, because people are addicted to nicotine, during the night when they are sleeping they do not smoke and can develop withdrawals from nicotine. When the body goes into withdrawal it is stressed due to not having something it has regularly, resulting in stress chemicals being released and wakefulness. Smoking also directly increases the stress response, as nicotine attaches to the receptors of the stress nervous system and releases stress chemicals, reducing the ability to sleep deeply.

Caffeine

Caffeine is the most commonly used mood-altering drug. Caffeine is a stimulant that activates the stress nervous system releasing several stress chemicals in the brain (including adrenaline and noradrenaline). Caffeine can improve concentration and give you a feeling of wellbeing. Caffeine improves athletic performance, improving both speed and power. Caffeine can also cause insomnia, anxiety, panic attacks and increase blood pressure depending on the dose and the sensitivity of the person.

Caffeine is addictive and withdrawal can occur. In people who have a daily coffee or tea at breakfast, if they abstain for 24 hours, 50 percent will develop a headache, a symptom of caffeine withdrawal. Personally, I have a large brewed cup of tea to get me going in the morning and on some mornings if I do not have my cuppa, I have experienced this caffeine withdrawal headache.

Caffeine is found naturally in more than 60 plants including coffee, tea, cola nut, cacao pod and guarana. Once consumed, caffeine appears in the blood stream within 30 to 60 minutes and is still present in the blood stream up to six hours later. The amount of caffeine varies in our drinks. A cup of coffee can have between 30 mg to 200 mg of caffeine. A cup of tea has approximately 30 mg of caffeine and 40 mg if the tea is brewed. A serving of dark chocolate can contain similar amounts of caffeine to a cup of tea. Popular tablets that people take to keep them awake, such as No-Doz, contain 100 to 200 mg of caffeine and cans of energy drink contain between 60 and 100 mg in total. Weight loss supplements can also contain large amounts of caffeine. The average daily intake is estimated to be 300 mg in developed countries. Coffee is big business and is second only to oil in the cost of imports to the United States.

Adding caffeine to products makes them taste better and people prefer the caffeinated version of most beverages. In the United States nearly 70 percent of all soft drinks contain caffeine. Soft drink manufacturers put caffeine into a wide range of soft drinks including root beer, orange soda, cream soda and lemon lime drinks (Mellow Yellow) to improve sales.[29]

People with insomnia, anxiety and depression are more likely to be sensitive to caffeine as they have a wound-up stress nervous system and release more stress chemicals for any stimulant. People with anxiety disorders are likely to experience episodes of anxiety or panic attacks at lower doses. Even in people without anxiety, taking 200 mg of caffeine can cause anxiety and higher doses can cause a panic attack.

Caffeine causes wakefulness with higher doses causing greater disruptions in sleep. Caffeine taken immediately before bedtime delays sleep onset, reduces total sleep time, alters the normal stages of sleep and decreases sleep quality. Even large doses of 200 mg taken at seven in the morning have been shown to disturb sleep; however, lower doses found in a cup of tea or coffee consumed in the morning do not usually affect sleep. A few studies have shown improvement in sleep duration and quality after complete abstinence from caffeine.

Caffeine is a stimulant, so it would be wise to restrict caffeinated drinks after midday, especially if you have trouble sleeping, otherwise caffeine will remain in your body and stimulate your mind when you are trying to get to sleep. Caffeine also aggravates anxiety and high doses should be avoided if you experience anxiety.

CHAPTER 10

MENOPAUSE

The menopause is a time in a woman's life where she no longer has a cyclic regular pattern of hormone release. The ovaries that have been so dependable since menstruation start to falter around the age of 50. Menstruation becomes irregular until it stops altogether. Menopause is said to occur once menstruation has stopped for one year.

As with any regular medication or hormone, once the regular supply becomes haphazard or stops altogether the body goes into a withdrawal. This withdrawal is accompanied by an activation of the stress nervous system that may explain several menopausal symptoms such as poor sleep and altered mood. It must be remembered that prior to the start of menopause insomnia, anxiety and depression can be present in up to a third of the population and menopause can be thought of as a stress that can aggravate insomnia, anxiety and depression, especially in those that already have a wound-up stress nervous system.

One of the most common symptoms around menopause is hot flushes – short periods of intense heat, often disturbing sleep. Oestrogen promotes dilation of blood vessels and when the body becomes warm blood vessels dilate in the skin to dissipate heat. With the reduced oestrogen the dilation of blood vessels is reduced, and heat is not dissipated as efficiently. This may be a factor leading to "hot flushes" during the menopause. These hot flushes can last for many years after the menopause. Reducing room temperature during menopause helps reduce sleep disturbance from hot flushes. Water filled blankets that can be set on cooling mode may be useful to reduce temperature while sleeping.

To alleviate the symptoms of menopause several strategies are promoted. One is to restore the hormones by taking hormone replacement therapy. Taking oestrogen tablets rapidly reduces the symptoms of menopause in the majority of women. Hormone replacement therapy was very popular until 2002 when a study was highly publicised showing a 29 percent increased risk of heart disease and 26 percent increased risk of breast cancer.[34] However, subsequent reviews of the data have shown hormone replacement therapy with oestrogen alone has no increased risk of breast cancer, and hormone replacement therapy with both oestrogen and progesterone has very small increases in risks of breast cancer. When prescribed before the age of 60 there is also no increased risk of heart disease. Hormones are also available in patches and these reduce the risk of all unwanted effects even more. Overall, current consensus is that hormone replacement therapy is very successful in improving menopausal symptoms and benefits outweigh the risks. It is not, however, recommended for women who have had breast cancer.

Insomnia, anxiety and depression that occur around menopause will respond to therapies that wind down the stress nervous system as discussed later in this book. A study performed by the University of Massachusetts Medical School showed Mindfulness based stress reduction improves the quality of life, sleep quality, anxiety, and stress at the menopause.[35] Other studies have shown yoga,[36] massage[37] and regular exercise[38] improve menopause-related insomnia.

A range of medications have been tried for menopausal symptoms. Paroxetine, an antidepressant, has been tested for hot flushes by both Georgetown University in the District of Columbia and University of Michigan and found to reduce hot flushes by around 50 percent. Paroxetine gained Federal Drug Agency approval in the United States for menopausal symptoms.[39,40] Many supplements claim to cure menopausal symptoms and are promoted with very few being subjected to rigorous scientific testing. Omega three supplements have been tested in a large trial of menopausal women and found to have no beneficial effect on menopausal symptoms of hot flushes, poor sleep or mood.[41]

CHAPTER 11

WHY AM I TIRED?

Fatigue is a feeling of tiredness that can develop due to several medical conditions and as a result of poor sleep. To understand fatigue that develops from poor sleep we need to look at the hormone cortisol which is a stress hormone released by the adrenal gland. Cortisol can surge in the blood after any stressful event such as an argument or public speaking. Once it is released you can often end up feeling on edge or keyed up. Trauma and surgery can also increase cortisol levels.

As well as being released by stress, cortisol also has a natural daily pattern with the highest levels in the early morning prior to waking, decreasing during the day down to almost zero in the late evening. Cortisol gives us energy, the high morning cortisol accounts for people feeling "like a box of birds", and the low levels at night create a feeling of sleepiness.

When we sleep, cortisol is produced slowly during the first six hours and much more quickly in the final two hours of sleep. Half of the total cortisol is released in the last two hours of sleep. It is like we wake with a battery at full charge. If sleep is disturbed and you wake before six hours of sleep you will miss out on the surge of cortisol in the last two hours of sleep.

As cortisol levels are highest in the morning, this is when people experiencing fatigue will have their highest levels of energy. Therefore, I often advise them to exercise or do activities in the morning rather than wait until the afternoon when they can feel too tired to exercise.

So, if we do not have enough cortisol in the morning we may feel tired. What happens if we have an excess of cortisol in the late evening? We have difficulty getting to sleep and sometimes wake in the middle of the night and can't get back to sleep. In one study researchers placed a dozen people with insomnia and a dozen people who slept well in a sleep laboratory for four nights.[42] Their sleep was monitored and their levels of cortisol were measured. They found people with insomnia produced greater amounts of total cortisol over 24 hours. Furthermore, they found stronger elevations in the late evening and early hours of the morning to around 3 am. This explains the difficulty getting to sleep as the brain is active often thinking about the day's events or worries ("chatty mind"). This also explains the early morning waking that occurs around 2 am.

When cortisol rises above a certain threshold, you will feel awake. Normally this threshold is reached around six to eight hours after falling asleep. If the cortisol level is elevated when you go to sleep, once cortisol production starts during sleep, the levels will increase above the wakeful threshold several hours earlier causing you to wake at 2 to 3 am and make you feel wide awake, creating difficulties getting back to sleep.

You may have heard the term adrenal fatigue. The extreme fatigue experienced in chronic insomnia, anxiety, depression and chronic fatigue syndrome is due to burnout of the adrenal gland with shrinking of the cells producing cortisol. Once this occurs the adrenal gland no longer produces as much cortisol overnight and you can wake with fatigue and be tired most of the day.

Researchers at Kings College London, Institute of Psychiatry investigated cortisol at seven different times of the day in 24 young people with chronic fatigue syndrome and compared this to 24 people who did not experience chronic fatigue.[43] Cortisol output during the day was significantly lower for people with chronic fatigue. After six months of treatment, they found cortisol levels increased to normal levels with a return of energy.

Over the past decade, I have seen many patients with chronic fatigue syndrome who have restored sleep, and over three to six months found their energy has returned. People first notice they wake occasionally with energy and then as months go on they wake more often with energy until finally they wake regularly like a "box of birds".

The cortisol rhythm is unaffected by short term sleep deprivation, prolonged bed rest or working one night shift.[44] After five nights of working night shift the circadian rhythm starts adjusting to the new time schedule.[45] The cortisol rhythm is upset by major shifts in time zone such as when travelling overseas. The reason jet lag occurs is due to the release of cortisol being out of sync with the time zone. If you travel around the globe where day is night, your cortisol will be highest towards the evening and lowest in the morning. Once you reach a new destination, it takes nearly a week for the pattern of cortisol secretion to adapt to the new time zone. Only time can adjust the body clock despite the numerous claims for products to help jet lag.

CHAPTER 12

ANXIETY

Anxiety is something we've all experienced from time to time and is essentially another word for worry. It is like having a police car with sirens ablaze behind you in the rear-view mirror as you are driving, thinking you've done something wrong when in fact most of the time the flashing lights have nothing to do with you and the police car sails past you. When people have excess fear or worry this is diagnosed as an anxiety disorder.

Panic attacks are common for people who experience anxiety. This is when you experience an intense, overwhelming attack of anxiety complete with sweating, fast pounding heartbeat, trembling, shortness of breath and shaking and thumping heart. Sometimes during a panic attack, you may feel you are going to collapse, lose control or die.

When patients with panic disorder were studied they were found to have increased activity of the stress nervous system compared to people without panic attacks.[42] Panic attacks can be associated with a range of conditions – anxiety, depression, bipolar disorder, eating disorders, obsessive-compulsive disorders, personality disorders, psychotic disorders and substance use disorders as well as many medical conditions.

As discussed in previous chapters, excess electricity can give rise to migraine symptoms, epilepsy attacks and insomnia. As we learned, the amygdala is the part of the brain that is involved in emotions, survival instincts and memory and is activated when a person experiences fear or aggression and is the primary area of the brain responsible for the fight or flight response. Excess electricity in the amygdala is one factor responsible for anxiety and panic attacks, and excess electricity in the amygdala may explain anger and irritability that often accompanies stress.

The stress nervous system that releases six stress chemicals into the brain has attachments to the amygdala and increases electricity. This part of the brain is likely to wind up and become exquisitely sensitive to normal everyday stimuli. Insomnia and depression are also symptoms produced by an overactive stress nervous system so we would expect people who experience one of these symptoms to experience the other symptoms. This is exactly what we find in the research.

People with general anxiety disorder are at increased risk of other diagnoses related to elevated stress nervous system activity. A quarter of the people with general anxiety disorder will also have a current diagnosis of social anxiety disorder or panic disorder. Nearly half will have a current diagnosis of depression. The lifetime risk of developing social anxiety disorder, panic disorder, low mood and major depression is up to 90 percent for people with generalised anxiety disorder.[47] A person is also likely to have more than one of these diagnoses at any time.

Anxiety disorders have been categorised as general anxiety disorder, social anxiety disorder and panic disorder. Generalised anxiety disorder is excessive worry about a variety of events or activities and interferes with everyday life. General anxiety disorder affects up to five percent of the population and up to 10 percent of women over 35 years of age. Reports suggest fewer than 20 percent of sufferers have a remission of symptoms.[48]

Social anxiety disorder is a marked fear of social situations in which the person feels scrutinised by others. Approximately 12 percent of the population will experience social anxiety disorder in their lifetime.[49] When exposed to social situations, the person fears he or she will be negatively judged as anxious, weak, crazy, stupid, boring, intimidating, dirty or unlikable. They are also concerned their actions, such as blushing, trembling, sweating, stumbling over their words, or staring, will be criticised by others.

Although labelled differently, general anxiety disorder, social anxiety and panic attacks are all a result of a wound-up stress nervous system that is designed to be anxious when faced with physical threats in the wild to ensure survival of the fittest. Unfortunately, what ensured survival of the fittest in the wild can cripple an individual in today's changing world.

CHAPTER 13

DEPRESSION

Life is a journey that requires significant navigation skills. No matter how skilled you are at navigating your way through this journey events happen that are often beyond your control. Death of a loved one, a romantic breakup, loss of a job, accidents, disability and taxes are unavoidable, and sadness is consequently a part of life. I sometimes wonder why we are all not a little depressed most of the time.

As I pointed out in earlier chapters insomnia, anxiety and depression are often found together as stress chemicals activate several parts of the brain simultaneously. In depression excess electricity is often present in the reticular formation (accounting for symptoms of poor sleep) and the amygdala (accounting for symptoms of anxiety and panic attacks). Changes in the hypothalamus are also present that also predispose to changes in appetite, energy and our 24-hour body clock.

While generally, electricity increases in insomnia and anxiety, in some parts of the brain electricity can reduce, leading to slowed thinking and movements in depression. In some parts of the brain when stress chemicals bombard them relentlessly they can switch off, rather than continue to create excess electricity. A reduction in electricity is likely to explain the slowness that accompanies some of the symptoms of depression.

The tide of depression seems to be ever increasing and reflects the ballooning number of antidepressant prescriptions being written by New Zealand doctors. The number of prescriptions written for all New Zealanders nearly doubled between 1997 and 2005. In this interval of only eight years, prescriptions of antidepressants increased from 1.1 million to 2.1 million.[50] In teenagers aged between 10 and 17 the number of prescriptions written increased by 44 percent in only four years from 2010 to 2014.

From 2008 to 2013, there was a 20 percent increase in the number of patients prescribed antidepressants. More than 400,000 people in New Zealand were prescribed antidepressants in 2013.[51] With a population of around four million in 2013 this represents more than one in 10 people taking antidepressants, remembering that the population includes babies and young children who are not usually prescribed this type of medication. The increase in antidepressant prescribing may not only reflect increasing numbers of people becoming depressed but also reflect a population more willing to take tablets and doctors more willing to prescribe them.

The average length of time a person becomes depressed has been found to be six months for the majority of people.[52] People experiencing a new episode of depression were followed to see who improved. The researchers found 50 percent of people recovered within three months, 75 percent within 12 months and 20 percent of people remain depressed when surveyed two years later.[53] Another study performed in the Netherlands showed an even bleaker result – 250 people diagnosed with depression were followed for two years and 60 percent experienced an ongoing depression at two years.[54]

The research paints a rather bleak picture for people who experience major depression. The research shows depression is more of a lifelong problem rather than just a temporary symptom. If a person experiences an episode of major depression, there is a 50 percent chance they will experience another episode in the following year, and the average number of times a person will experience depression during their lifetime is 13.[55]

Compounding the poor outcomes for people with depression is the fact that our current first-line treatment antidepressants tablets do not work as well as we would hope. One such study of over 2,500 people performed in 41 centres looked into how many of the patients achieved a remission (their depression subsided) when prescribed the antidepressant Citalopram. Only 30 percent of people achieved a remission.[56]

Research has shown the number of people who

become depressed varies in different parts of the world. In the United States five percent of the population were in a state of depression during the survey and 17 percent of the population experienced depression at sometime during their lifetime.[57] Another study measured depression in five different countries in Europe, measuring both city and rural centres in each country. There was a wide variation in depression with rates for depression reaching 15 percent in Liverpool while in Santander, Spain only 1.8 percent of the population were depressed. In a rural site in the United Kingdom only five percent of people were depressed as opposed to 15 percent in Liverpool city.[58] Climate differences between Liverpool and Santander may help explain some of the differences in depression rates as heat reduces the activity of the stress nervous system. The increased stress of living in cities as opposed to the countryside may explain the variation between the city and country rates of depression.

Students are at high risk of depression. As well as coping with financial hardship they also have the stress of deadlines for assignments and exams. The double edge sword around exams that makes students prone to these symptoms is that high levels of concentration release stress chemicals as well as stress regarding passing exams. They often study for long hours prior to exams and have reduced time to perform activities such as exercise that reduces stress chemicals. Medical students have been studied and found to have depression rates of 30 percent, almost three times more than the rest of the population.[59]

Samantha, a university student, came to see me in 2015 after she dropped out of university. In October, while studying for exams, she was having difficulty sleeping. She was having difficulty falling asleep, often taking hours to get to sleep. She would then wake in the early hours of the morning with difficulty returning to sleep.

Anxiety was also creeping in about whether she would pass exams. She kept worrying about her courses, financial situation and even questioned what she was doing at university. She stopped running or going to the gym. Even on a Friday night she could not drag herself out to socialise with friends and noticed her social world shrinking as she became more isolated. She lost her appetite and started losing weight at almost a kilogram a week.

Samantha decided to stop university and fly home. Out of the pressure cooker environment of university exams she immediately felt she could gather her thoughts. She started an antidepressant, exercising regularly and attending the sauna at her local swimming pool. She connected with friends and family and over the next few months started sleeping well and returning to her usual self. After several months off she returned to university the following year to complete her studies. A spiral of symptoms occurs once the stress nervous system winds up with poor sleep, reduced exercise and isolation. Disturbed sleep leading to poor energy and depression can quickly derail your life.

CHAPTER 14

THE ROLE OF STRESS IN DEPRESSION

First lifetime episodes of depression are typically more related to major life stresses than subsequent episodes. With each episode of depression, lower levels of stress are required to precipitate another episode of depression.[60] With each episode of depression, the stress nervous system becomes wound tighter and releases more stress chemicals for any given stress making it easier to develop depression in the future.

Several researchers have shown children who experience stressful events, such as parental loss or physical abuse, are more likely to develop depression as adults.[61,62,63] A study performed by The University of Los Angeles, California followed young women for two years and correlated the development of depression with the levels of stress they experienced.[61] They found young women exposed to childhood trauma developed depression with lower levels of stressful events.

Women are twice as likely to develop depression.[64] This may be partly explained by women producing a third more stress chemicals than men for the same given stress. Research has also shown that major stressful life events are more common for females than males, especially in the 10 to 19-year old age group.[61] Social support protects people from the effects of stress and losing your social support increases depression, thus higher rates are found in people who divorce or separate than those who are married.[65]

Over a decade ago I saw Craig who was 40 years old. When he presented to me there was a mismatch. He presented as a mild mannered, pleasant man who brought along his daughter to the consultation. His notes, however, showed a very different picture. He had an unsettling past and suffered from headache, migraine, insomnia, irritability and anger. He had poor impulse control as well as severe depression. Craig had been under the care of psychiatrists for over a decade and despite several antidepressant medications, counselling and psychotherapy, he had made several suicide attempts. His home life was troubled and he was divorced from his wife and had one 10-year-old daughter.

Craig worked as a roofing contractor and a few years prior he tried to commit suicide. This time he fired a nail gun into his head and lived to tell the tale. The most surprising thing that happened once he recovered was a complete change in his character. He became a mild mannered friendly and pleasant person. He was no longer aggressive and irritable. He slept well and was no longer depressed. He no longer went to the psychiatrist or any other person for treatment of his mood. I found it hard to believe what had happened. It was like a miracle. Craig shot the part of his brain that helps orchestrate the production of stress chemicals. He no longer produced stress chemicals such as adrenaline or cortisol in response to stress. In 30 years of dealing with patients this is the only time I have come across this story and it strengthened my belief about stress and the development of insomnia, anxiety and depression.

CHAPTER 15

HOW ARE PEOPLE WITH DEPRESSION DIFFERENT?

In the last few months of writing this book I talked to several doctors with over 30 years' experience and posed the question – are there structural differences in people who experience depression and people who are not depressed? All of them remarked they had never heard of any differences between people who experienced depression when compared to people without depression. Before I started this book I was also unaware of any structural differences. After taking a close look at the research, to my fascination, I found several structural differences in people who experience depression.

The hypothalamus in the brain is a finely tuned thermostat that maintains a balance of several body functions such as appetite, sleep, temperature and daily rhythms. The fine tuning of the hypothalamus is often upset in people with depression. Some individuals have reduced appetite with weight loss while other people can increase their appetite and gain weight. Some people experience difficulty sleeping while other people can sleep more than usual. Early morning waking with difficulty getting back to sleep is common. Sexual interest or desire can also reduce. Agitation (inability to sit still, pacing) can be present or slowed speech and body movements can develop. Decreased energy, fatigue, difficulty thinking, concentrating and making decisions are often present.

The hypothalamus activates the pituitary gland in the brain, which in turn activates the adrenal gland to produce the stress chemicals cortisol, adrenaline and noradrenaline that are released into the bloodstream and spread throughout the body. Many factors point to a wound up and enlarged stress nervous system being a significant factor in causing depression.

Firstly, researchers at Washington University School of Medicine and Harvard University showed the activity of the stress nervous system is elevated in depressed individuals when compared to individuals that are not depressed by measuring heart rate variability.[62] Researchers in Germany had similar conclusions and found the activity of the stress nervous system reduces when depression is treated successfully.[67]

Researchers from the Neurosciences Research Center, Medical College of Pennsylvania and Harbor-UCLA Medical Center in California measured adrenal size by MRI scan in people with and without depression. The adrenal gland was found to be 70 percent larger in people who were depressed.[68] The good news is once depression is successfully treated the adrenal gland returns to normal size.

Another group of researchers at Duke University Medical Center in North Carolina measured the pituitary gland by MRI scan in 20 people experiencing major depression and 39 people without depression.[69] They found the pituitary gland was 30 percent larger in people with depression. Furthermore the research has found a 52 percent reduction in GABA levels (Chapter 5) and a 19 percent reduction in the size of the hippocampus (Chapter 17), an important memory centre of the brain, for people with major depression.

What does this mean for people with depression? The research shows the parts of the brain and body responsible for the stress response grow and produce more stress chemicals during everyday life and for any given stressor, perpetuating their risk of symptoms for decades. Fortunately the structural and physiological changes that occur are all reversible with the solutions discussed later in this book.

CHAPTER 16

THE BABY BLUES

Having a new baby is a special event but at the same time often fraught with difficulty. It can be stressful as it may be a new experience requiring significant adjustment. The thing many parents remember is the lousy sleep. The frequent disturbances to feed the baby and sometimes inexplicable waking of a baby can leave most parents in a daze.

The sleep disturbance can often last up to 12 months and often beyond for the most unfortunate. When women have been asked about their sleep disturbance in studies they described their sleep disturbance as extreme, resulting in exhaustion and causing them to lose patience with their partners.[70] Post-partum sleep disturbance is associated with poor quality of life, decreased concentration and lack of general wellbeing and affects the infant, the mum and the family. It is also a serious risk factor for depression.

To answer the questions of whether hormones or poor sleep was the factor that resulted in post-partum depression, a study was performed by the University of Pittsburgh, School of Medicine where pregnant women were followed from 36 weeks pregnant until well after the baby was born.[71] At the start of the study none of the pregnant woman was depressed. Questionnaires to measure their sleep and depression were carried out as well as a psychiatrist interview.

Blood tests were performed at regular intervals to measure the changes in hormone levels during late pregnancy and after delivery. They measured prolactin, cortisol and oestradiol. Within 17 weeks of delivery, 20 percent of the women became depressed. Both hormone scores and sleep scores changed significantly over the study period. The analyses showed the levels of hormones did not correlate with the development of depression. Only sleep scores predicted the onset of depression. For every one point increase in sleep disturbance women were 25 percent more at risk of developing depression.

The article summarised that poor sleep quality during the first 17 weeks after delivery was associated with the development of depression while changes in hormones had no significant effect on mood. This highlights the importance of sleep deprivation on mood. To prevent post-partum depression, mothers need support around the birth to ensure they have a break at night from feeding the baby. New mums also need time to exercise or do activities that will promote sleep.

CHAPTER 17

DEPRESSION AND DEMENTIA, LOSING YOUR MIND

Depression can lead to poor memory and concentration. In the elderly this can commonly be confused with a diagnosis of dementia. The hippocampus is a part of the brain that is important to memory. Studies over the past three decades have shown the hippocampus shrinks in people with dementia compared to people without dementia.[72] There is also a natural shrinking of this part of the brain with ageing that may explain the increase in dementia as we age. In the 65 to 69 age group seven people in every 1,000 develop dementia while in the 80 to 85 age group this increases to 118 people in every 1,000 people.[73]

During the stress response corticotrophin releasing hormone attaches to several parts of the brain important to memory including the hippocampus and may be one factor explaining the poor memory and concentration that accompany most stress related disorders including insomnia, anxiety and depression. "Brain fog" is often the term used to describe this phenomenon.

Researchers have measured the size of the hippocampus with MRI scans in people with stress related conditions with uniform findings, a reduction in the size of the hippocampus. Researchers from Emory University School of Medicine in Atlanta and Yale University School of Medicine, compared hippocampus volume in women with childhood sexual abuse and post-traumatic stress disorder and women without abuse or post-traumatic stress disorder. They found a 19 percent reduction in hippocampus volume in women with childhood abuse and post-traumatic stress disorder.[74]

Freiburg University Medical Centre, Freiburg, Germany performed MRI scans on a group of people with chronic insomnia and a group of people without insomnia, showing a reduction in hippocampus size for people with chronic insomnia.[75] People who are depressed were also found to have reduced hippocampus volume compared to people who are not depressed.[76,77]

It seems any prolonged activation of the stress nervous system as occurs in post-traumatic stress disorder, insomnia, anxiety and depression reduces hippocampus volume and predisposes to poor memory. This may hasten the onset of dementia as we age. The best way to find out if depression increases our chance of dementia is to follow a large group of the population over a few decades and see how many depressed people develop dementia and compare this with people who are not depressed.

In the Netherlands 3,000 depressed people over the age of 55 were followed from 1993 until 2014, a total of 21 years. The researchers performed surveys at three different points from 1993 to 2004 and tracked participants' depression levels over these three time points.[78] In 2014 they looked at who developed dementia. In people who experienced persistent depression the risk of developing dementia doubled. The research showed people who were depressed in 1993 and improved at subsequent follow–ups were not at significantly increased risk of dementia.

A study following people with anxiety also found people had twice the risk of developing dementia.[79] The stress response is widespread and when it continues unchecked for prolonged periods may accelerate the onset of dementia.

So far, we have looked at the doom and gloom of excess stress. We have looked at the possible cause of stress related disorders starting with a wind-up of the stress nervous system components due to prolonged stress or trauma such as in childhood or in adulthood. Once the parts of the brain and body producing stress chemicals grow and our natural off switch in the brain shrinks, we become prone to symptoms being present for many years. Now we will look at the solutions for insomnia, anxiety and depression.

CHAPTER 18

SOLUTIONS THAT CAN HELP

Life stressors are inevitable, they come in all shapes and sizes with some taking a few days and others taking months or years to deal with. Prolonged stress results in the stress nervous system becoming more sensitive and winding up like a spring. Combined with a loss of our brain "off switch", this leads to a lifelong pattern of symptoms that include insomnia, anxiety and depression. The solution must target the cause – unwind the stress nervous system and restore the neurons in the brain that act as an off switch.

The research shows exercise, sauna, meditation/ breathing, yoga and Tai Chi performed a minimum of three to five times a week over three to four months unwind the stress nervous system. Each time you perform one of these activities you unwind the stress nervous system a little. If performed once a week the stress nervous system will unwind a little, but the week's stresses will wind it up again. If performed repeatedly during the week the stress nervous system unwinds a little each time and does not have the chance to wind up again.

Many techniques that calm the stress nervous system

are based on feedback. For example, danger activates the stress nervous system leading to fast breathing. Slow breathing signals that there is no danger, so the stress nervous system calms down. Danger leads to the stress nervous system shunting all the blood to the muscles required for fighting or running and constricting blood vessels in the hands and feet leading to cold hands and feet (a sign of an overactive stress nervous system). Heat dilates blood vessels, sending signals back to the brain to reduce the output of stress chemicals.

Activities that reduce stress nervous system activity work in two ways. The first is to calm the stress nervous system as occurs in deep breathing, yoga, meditation and Tai Chi. The second way is to activate the stress nervous system with activities that result in the depletion of stress chemicals. Moderate exercise to where you become a little breathless (above 50 percent maximum heart rate) and sauna bathing both increase stress nervous system activity; however, the stress chemicals are quickly depleted by the exercise and sweating so the stress chemical cycle is completed. Repeatedly performing moderate exercise and sauna reduce the overall activity of the stress nervous system.

When someone experiences insomnia, anxiety or depression their brain is wound up and is having difficulty coping with daily life. It becomes very difficult to process underlying trauma, change their psychological outlook or their social world. Once the stress nervous system is unwound the mind is more receptive to work through underlying psychological trauma through counselling, psychological therapies or mindfulness. Once the brain is unwound you can also examine faulty thinking patterns such as catastrophising (always thinking the worst thing will happen), self-talk such as you are not good enough or other factors that are perpetuating your symptoms. Over time you can help change thinking patterns that will hold you back from living an enjoyable and fulfilling life with a deep sense of joy. With a clear mind you can also take stock of your life and eliminate those things that cause you stress. You can also start returning to hobbies and social activities that you once enjoyed.

In June 2018 I discovered from research papers that GABA levels are reduced in the brain in people with insomnia, anxiety and depression. This neurotransmitter has an almost opposite action to stress neurotransmitters, GABA reduces electricity in the brain and acts as an off switch. The research shows meditation is likely to restore the GABA levels to improve insomnia, anxiety and depression. The exact dose to reverse these changes in the brain is unknown but from my reading 40 minutes of meditation or slow breathing per day for three months is likely to increase GABA levels.

I always wondered why I was prone to poor sleep

intermittently despite having good exercise habits. I suspect that the neurons producing GABA that suppress electricity have never been allowed to return to normal function. I started meditating one hour per day while on holiday. I set my timer on for 20 minutes and try to perform three sessions in a row. I suspect by regularly performing meditation this part of my brain will expand and improve my sleep habits in the future.

CHAPTER 19

WHY SHOULD I EXERCISE?

We are animals by design who have mastered our world to a certain extent that resigns many of us to sedentary lives. People need to realise that regular exercise is not just a "good idea" but depletes stress chemicals and is a long-term cure for insomnia, anxiety and depression.

Moderate exercise (above 50 percent maximum heart rate) stresses the body creating the release of stress chemicals throughout the brain and body.[80] Subsequently the elevated stress chemicals are depleted by exercise, completing the stress chemical cycle and leaving an individual relaxed. The medical research shows people who exercise regularly have reduced stress nervous system activity compared to people who do not exercise regularly. [81]

Multiple studies show performing regular exercise reduces the activity of your stress nervous system.[82,83,84] The Karolinska Hospital, Karolinska Institute in Stockholm, Sweden showed 50 minutes three times a week maintaining heart rate at over 50 percent heart rate maximum for eight weeks reduced the activity of the stress nervous system.[82] The 50 minute programme consisted of a variety of exercises performed for three or four minutes such as walking, jogging, flexibility and strength training of the large muscles. The programme was accompanied by music.

Researchers from Seattle Veterans Affairs Medical Center and the University of Washington, Seattle showed 45 minutes walking or cycling four to five times a week over six months improved heart rate variability that measures stress nervous system activity by 68 percent.[83] A research collaboration from Columbia, Chile and Spain tested medium intensity exercise and high intensity exercise on sedentary individuals.[84] Both groups exercised three times a week over 12 weeks. The medium intensity group walked fast or jogged on a treadmill for 15 to 55 minutes while the fast intensity group sprinted four minutes with four minutes reduced intensity exercise, repeating this four times. Both groups had significant reductions in activity of their stress nervous systems.

CHAPTER 20

EXERCISE FOR INSOMNIA AND ANXIETY

So far, we know the activity of the stress nervous system is elevated in people who experience insomnia, anxiety and depression. Now we have found out exercise reduces the activity of the stress nervous system. The next question is whether exercise will reverse the symptoms of insomnia, anxiety and depression.

The exercise research for insomnia and anxiety are in their infancy with fewer trials performed, with far more studies performed for depression. The next few chapters present the research and are detailed enough to leave you in no doubt that exercise is an extremely important weapon to treat insomnia, anxiety and depression. Over the past three decades I have maintained an exercise regime that has varied over the decades in terms of activities but I have never exercised less than three times a week in all this time. I am sure this is one of the reasons I have personally experienced no recurrences of depression in three decades.

Moderate exercise unwinds the stress nervous system and improves sleep. Even a single episode of exercise consisting of running on a treadmill (10 minutes three times with a 10 minute break in between) reduced time to get to sleep by 55 percent and increased total sleep time by 18 percent.[85] Moderate aerobic exercise was tested for people with long term insomnia. Participants used a treadmill three times a week for 50 minutes for six months.[86] People in the exercise group increased their total sleep time by 1.4 hours from 4.8 hours to 6.2 hours and their time to get to sleep reduced from one hour to 26 minutes on average.

Researchers at Stanford University compared mindfulness-based stress reduction and exercise for social anxiety disorder. The exercise group were given a gym membership for two months and advised to exercise three times a week. Both groups showed significant reductions in anxiety and depression that remained for three months after the eight weeks of exercise.[87] Another trial performed at the University of Amsterdam in the Netherlands compared mindfulness-based stress reduction, exercise on a spin bike and abdominal breathing for young adults who were experiencing stress.[88] Participants performed daily practice for five weeks, initially five minutes per day for the first week, 10 minutes for the next week and 20 minutes daily for the last three weeks. All groups improved their mindfulness, self-compassion and worry equally.

What about combinations, will they help any

more than exercise alone? A study by researchers at University Health Systems of Eastern Carolina and the University of Massachusetts tested this proposition.[89] People who experienced anxiety were placed into three groups. One group performed exercise alone, another group performed exercise and cognitive behavioural therapy and the last group had no treatment. Jogging or running was performed for 20 minutes three times a week for six weeks. The exercise group and combination of exercise and cognitive behavioural therapy both had significant reductions in anxiety with the no treatment group having minimal improvement. In the short term it seems exercise alone is enough to improve anxiety. The great thing about this study is that exercise does not have to be expensive and is available to most people. Going to therapy is expensive and out of reach for many people living in the western world.

At the Free University of Berlin exercise has also been tested for panic attacks.[86] The effect of a single bout of treadmill exercise at 70 percent of maximum heart rate for 30 minutes was tested for chemical induced panic attacks. Subjects were given a chemical known to induce panic attacks after a period of rest and after exercise on the treadmill. The exercise group experienced half the number of panic attacks than the group who did not exercise. The next chapter will examine the effectiveness of exercise for depression.

CHAPTER 21

EXERCISE, THE CURE FOR DEPRESSION

A multitude of studies have investigated exercise for depression and found both aerobic and weights-based programmes three to four times a week for eight weeks can improve depression. Exercise has been compared to psychotherapy, antidepressants and cognitive therapy and found to be just as effective, in fact long term follow-up shows exercise is superior to antidepressants. I have highlighted trials which are around eight weeks long as this is the time frame required to reduce the activity of the stress nervous system.

To investigate the best dose of exercise for depression, researchers from Colorado, Texas and Alberta, Canada compared low dose exercise and moderate exercise (Public Health Dose – for example jogging, swimming, fast walking for 30 minutes daily) with a group that performed flexibility exercises for 12 weeks.[91] The groups were further separated into two groups. One performed the exercise dose three days a week while the other group exercised five days a week. The group performing moderate exercise experienced a far greater improvement in depression compared to the low dose exercise and flexibility exercise group.

This study highlighted a few more interesting facts. People who exercise three times a week and five times a week had similar responses as long as they performed a moderate level of exercise and expended the same amount of energy. At the start of the exercise all groups had an average Hamilton Rating Depression score of around 19 (on this scale greater than 17 is moderate to severe depression) and at the end of the study the average scores for the moderate exercise groups were under 10 (under 10 is not depressed). Many health professionals are sceptical of the ability of depressed people to attend exercise. In this study 80 percent of depressed participants managed to attend exercise three times a week for the duration of the study.

Psychiatrists in Norway studied the effect of aerobic exercise for patients with major depression who were admitted to a psychiatric hospital.[92] Patients performed moderate aerobic exercise (50 to 70 percent of maximum heart rate) one hour three times a week resulting in significant reductions in depression. The more a person's fitness improved the less depressed they became. They concluded that exercise had a significant antidepressant effect in patients admitted to hospital for depression.

Researchers at Wakayama Medical University, Japan, performed a trial of jogging five times a week for 50 minutes for young females aged between 18 and 20 with depression.[93] The group-based jogging began with 5 to 10 minutes warm-up, about 30 minutes jogging and 15 minutes warm-down. At the start of the study the average depression score was in the severe depression range and after the eight weeks the average score reduced into the non depressed range. In this study the researchers also measured stress chemicals including adrenaline and cortisol and found both reduced after eight weeks of exercise.

The following two studies comparing conventional antidepressant medication with exercise can really enlighten us on how effective exercise is for depression. A study of a university psychiatric clinic in Italy recruited females aged between 20 and 40 who failed to respond to antidepressants after two months.[94] Patients were randomised to either continuing antidepressants or adding exercise to their antidepressant regime. Patients were followed at two, four, six and eight months. The exercise consisted of two 60-minute sessions per week of warm up, strengthening on machines and stretching for eight months. At the start of the trial the patients in the exercise group were moderately and severely depressed (average scores on the Hamilton depression rating scale over 20). At the end of the study the exercise group had an average score of six meaning they were no longer depressed (under 10 means no depression). The group that continued antidepressants began with an average score of 19 and eight months later ended with an average score of 17 (greater than 17 is moderate to severe depression). After eight months the depression scores of the exercise group reduced 66 percent with the average plummeting into the non-depressed range while the antidepressant group scores reduced by 13 percent with average scores shifting very slightly.

Researchers at Duke University Medical Center, in North Carolina compared three treatments for depression – antidepressant alone, exercise alone and antidepressant plus exercise.[95] The antidepressant sertraline was prescribed for one group. One group performed aerobic exercise for 30 minutes three times a week at 70 percent of their heart rate maximum while a third group was assigned to an antidepressant and exercise. The trial ran for four months when measurements were taken. Measurements on participants were repeated at 10 months.

The researchers found 60 to 65 percent of all groups became non-depressed at four months. The next follow-up at ten months yielded very interesting results. At 10 months 70 percent of the exercise group remained depression free while 48 percent of those taking antidepressants were depression free and 45 percent of people using antidepressants and exercise were depression free. Of the people who responded to treatment at four months, only eight percent had relapsed into depression in the exercise group, while

38 percent relapsed in the antidepressant group and 31 percent relapsed in the exercise plus antidepressant group. The number of minutes per week a person exercised significantly predicted whether they would be depressed or not at the end of the study.

This trial showed that combining an antidepressant with exercise reduced the effectiveness of exercise to reduce depression at 10 months. An important question is why would taking an antidepressant stop the beneficial effects of exercise? A likely explanation why the antidepressant reduced the effectiveness of exercise at 10 months is because antidepressant medication increases the activity of the stress nervous system, counteracting the beneficial effects of exercise at 10 months.

Research in Sydney, Australia has looked into a gym-based weights programme as a treatment for depression. A trial looked at using weights machines three times a week for 45 minutes for ten weeks in the over 60 age group.[96] The exercises included chest press, lat pull downs, leg press, knee extension and knee flexion. Patients performed three sets of eight repetitions for 45 minutes duration. To establish their dose of weights, the maximum weight was the weight at which they could perform one lift and then 80 percent of this weight was used. The results were impressive with depression scores reducing by 60 percent. In fact, when I checked the scores, the average score on the

Beck Depression Inventory was 21 (over 20 is moderate depression) at the start of the study and after the exercise the average score was 9.8 (a score under 10 means there is no depression). Furthermore, 88 percent of the exercise group that had major depression no longer experienced major depression.

In another Australian study high intensity weight training has been compared to low intensity weight training for major depression using a variety of weight lifting machines found at most gyms.[97] Sixty people were randomised to high intensity weight training (80 percent maximum load), low intensity weight training (20 percent maximum load) and no exercise. Each exercise session lasted 60 minutes and was performed three times a week for eight weeks. Twice as many people who performed the high intensity weight training improved compared to low intensity weight training. When the Hamilton Depression Rating Scores are looked at, the average for the high intensity weight training group was 20 (moderate to severe depression) and after eight weeks the average reduced to 8.4 (less than 10 means a person has no depression).

Running has also been compared to weight lifting to treat depression at the University of Rochester, New York.[98] Forty people with an average of five episodes of previous depression were recruited and randomised to either running or weight lifting four times a week for eight weeks. The depression scores reduced significantly for both exercise groups and did not change for the group doing no exercise. At three months 82 percent of the running group and 79 percent of the weight lifting group were no longer depressed. Similar results continued at seven months.

Walking has been studied in randomised control trials for depression.[99] Most studies used small numbers and showed only slight improvements in depression for patients who were doing no physical activity at the start of the study. If you are performing zero physical activity then walking may be a good starting point to build physical stamina for more intense exercise. However, if you are already walking regularly and experiencing insomnia, anxiety or depression either switching to more vigorous exercise or changing to regular sauna bathing/ steam room or other therapies would be advisable.

While regular exercise can improve mood one study looked at the effects of stopping exercise for people who exercised regularly. People who exercised 30 minutes, three times a week, were advised to stop all exercise and followed for two weeks. The researchers found mood worsened in people who stopped exercising, as early as two weeks.[100]

The facts are clear. Regular exercise has benefits for insomnia, anxiety and depression. Regular exercise can improve up to 80 percent of people who have depression.

Exercise is an excellent option for people who experience depression and a regular exercise habit will prevent depression returning. Over the years I have counselled many patients to help them start an exercise habit. There are many barriers to exercise including time, pain and disability, motivation, fatigue and expense.

Time is often an issue with people due to work commitments, commuting and family demands. Not everyone can take himself or herself to the pool or gym. I often recommend people with time constraints to buy a piece of exercise equipment such as an exercycle or cross trainer and perform 20 minutes in front of the television three to four times a week. This saves travelling somewhere to exercise. Many patients have bought themselves a machine and successfully begun a regular exercise programme.

Many patients I see have difficulties doing exercise due to injuries and arthritic joints. Pressure on joints will often exacerbate pain. If someone has arthritis of the knee then jogging will usually exacerbate pain and in this situation a cycle or cross trainer may be better. People with low back pain often develop pain on sitting for long periods and using a cross trainer or treadmill would be better than rowing or cycling. Trial and error is often required. Try the activity and if it aggravates pain then try another activity.

I have significant changes in my lower back and

experienced two years of lower back pain. I was a keen kayaker but experienced pins and needles down both legs when I kayaked for over 10 minutes. I was also a keen cycler having participated in long cycle races of over 100 kilometres. Once I found out the state of my back I sold my kayaks and cycle. I mostly perform cross training or swimming as my main form of exercise as there is less pressure going through my spine.

For people with hip and knee pain I often advise going to the swimming pool and walking up and down the pool with water to waist or chest height for 20 to 40 minutes. This provides plenty of resistance and reduces impact on the joints due to the weightlessness experienced by being immersed in water. To lose weight many patients have attended the swimming pool 40 minutes five days a week and lost several kilograms of weight over six months. Many swimming pools also have sauna, steam rooms or spas, so after exercising you can relax in the heat.

If you experience fatigue, when starting an exercise habit start gently and build up the time and intensity gradually. Another sensible piece of advice is to exercise in the morning as this is the peak energy time for most people. The hormone that determines energy is always highest in the morning and lowest in the evenings. Expense can be avoided if you can learn an exercise programme that uses body weight and no equipment, or second hand equipment can often be bought cheaply.

As we are animals with reduced avenues for physical activity, one important role of exercise is to reduce stress chemicals enhancing our sleep and mood. In a world where significant factors compete for your time, it is important to look after yourself above all else. I find programming my time for exercise and sauna during the week works and if anyone wants me to do something at my designated exercise times I refuse (unless in extreme emergency situations). I often say to patients "what you do everyday will determine how you end up in two or three years or several decades time."

As many of us reach our 50s and 60s there is a lot at risk if we do not look after our minds and bodies. If we are not looking after our health we may look forward to a life in a nursing home for the elderly if we lose our mobility or senses. When I recommend exercise the minimum dose would be 20 to 30 minutes four times a week of exercise to the level where you feel slightly breathless. As a bonus, exercise has also been shown to reduce the risks of cancer, heart disease, diabetes, hypertension and disability as we age.

CHAPTER 22

THE MAGIC OF HEAT

Heat has been used for relaxation for many centuries. The Romans were famous for their bath houses. The Japanese have Sento and Onsen. Sauna bathing also forms an important part of many other cultures including the Finnish, Inuit and Native Americans.

It is a well-known fact that pain increases as the temperature plummets, the winter can certainly bring out those aches and pains. Furthermore, research shows populations that live in colder climates experience more pain compared to those in warmer climates. Headache and migraine are least common in Africa, intermediate in Asia and most common in Europe. Stress related illnesses follow a similar pattern. New Zealand has a very high rate of depression and suicide. Countries such as Fiji are famous for having a very relaxed population.

Wellington is officially the windiest city in the world, the wind sometimes escalating the cold significantly more than the mercury suggests. When I was a teenager my parents would take the family back to India for two to three months over the school holidays. The weather there was a constant 25 degrees. We have a house in a village and would play cricket in the street and visit the local city. I will never forget the feeling of being very relaxed after a few weeks of arriving due to the hot weather combined with the slow pace of life. However, I would return to Wellington and the feelings of relaxation would subside.

I found out how heat produces relaxation when I was studying for my PhD over a decade ago. I remember reading a book out of the medical library on hand warming for headache, something very unusual. You see, there are several medical trials showing hand warming helps tension headache. It took several years before I could explain this strange phenomenon. Increased activity of the stress nervous system constricts blood vessels in the hands, causing cold hands. By warming the hands you are dilating the blood vessels and sending messages back to the brain to reduce the activity of the stress nervous system. By warming hands using hot packs, hot water in the sink, wearing gloves in cold weather, rubbing the hands together vigorously or just holding a hot drink you can actually reduce the activity of the stress nervous system. Regular warming of the hands during the day will create an enduring sense of relaxation and reduce stress related symptoms over several months. The saying "cold hands warm heart" makes a lot of sense as those who worry about others release stress chemicals that result in cold hands.

I always enjoyed playing hockey, running and

swimming through my twenties and thirties. The exercise certainly helped me sleep better but the nightmares would still come. After learning about the effects of heat I started regular sauna bathing and attending hot yoga. After several months I felt more relaxed. The nightmares and night sweats also reduced significantly.

I felt my whole persona was unwinding, I was less uptight, worried less about money, and I felt free for the first time in my life. My new self started reading endless books on Buddhism, mindfulness, Tao Te Ching and books by Eckhart Tolle, Mahatma Gandhi and many others. My morality and spirituality were being awakened along with my mind being freed of excess worry that had plagued me in my everyday life.

The heat associated with variations in seasons is likely to explain why depression is worse in winter. A study done over four years relating depression to temperature, found that depression increased with reduced temperature.[101]

A study of depression rates around the world by one group of researchers using the same measurement tools found depression was six times greater in Liverpool, England than Santander, Spain.[56] I suspect this may be related to the warmer weather. The same study found Finland had a lower rate of depression and I wonder if this is due to the cultural habit of sauna bathing.

Utilising heat for stress related disorders sounds like

a great idea. A single episode of sauna bathing causes heat stress and creates exactly the same response as rigorous exercise, releasing adrenaline, noradrenaline and cortisol.[102,103,104] After 15 minutes in the sauna you can often feel your heart racing due to the increased adrenaline being released. The sauna completes the stress chemical cycle resulting in sweating and attending the sauna repeatedly calms the stress nervous system.

For people who cannot tolerate heat, gradual introduction of sauna bathing for five-minute intervals followed by a cold shower can help you cope with the heat. Alternatively with an infrared sauna you can set the temperature as low as 40 degrees and then increase it as you can tolerate the heat. People often ask if there is any benefit of infra-red sauna versus a charcoal sauna. Both are equally effective.

Several studies have been performed in Japan for something they have called Waon therapy – going into a sauna at 60 degrees for 15 minutes followed by lying down for 30 minutes. Several studies in Japan showed that performing Waon therapy five times a week for four weeks reduces the activity of the stress nervous system as measured by heart rate variability. The studies also showed Waon therapy reduces levels of stress chemicals adrenaline and noradrenaline after four weeks of therapy.[105,106,107]

A study at Hamamatsu University School of Medicine

in Japan investigated the effects of a single 20 to 30 minute sauna bathing session. They measured the response of 45 people before and after attending the sauna and found significant improvements in anxiety and depression scores.[108]

A study performed by Kagoshima University Hospital in Japan found Waon therapy, five times a week for four weeks, resulted in improvements in anxiety and depression.[109] Blood tests also showed a reduction in noradrenaline (stress chemical) after four weeks. Attending the sauna for two to three months is likely to lead to an even higher percentage of patients improving. For my PhD I performed a study where patients with daily tension-type headache attended the sauna for 20 minutes three times a week for eight weeks. The participants had endured headache symptoms for an average of 16 years. In this study 76 percent of patients in the sauna group had a marked reduction in their tension-type headache. Sleep improved 50 percent and depression scores also improved in the sauna group.[110]

The research on sauna bathing for stress related conditions is in its infancy and I hope more trials are performed over the coming years for insomnia, anxiety and depression. Sauna bathing is likely to be one of the best interventions for insomnia, anxiety and depression as it rapidly creates a sense of profound relaxation.

Daniel experienced poor sleep for 40 years and when

I asked, “What happened in your past?” (childhood) he said he could not recall anything bad happening. Daniel came from Scotland to New Zealand at age six with his parents and four siblings in 1972. His siblings were aged 4, 5, 7 and 8. His father was an alcoholic and spent the family money on alcohol. After a few years in New Zealand, his father returned to Scotland leaving his family behind. Both losing his father and being raised by a single mother with several children are likely to be the trauma that contributed to his poor sleeping patterns.

When I first met Daniel he was going to bed at 10 pm and taking a few hours to get to sleep. He had a chatty mind and could not get his mind to relax enough to fall asleep. Once asleep he would wake at four in the morning and often disturb his wife as he was unable to return to sleep. He also experienced night sweats, a sign of an overactive stress nervous system. The erratic pattern of sleep meant he was very tired during the day. He worked as an electrician and luckily he was self-employed as he would pull over to the side of the road or car park and have a nap most days due to his exhaustion. Despite his fatigue he tried to keep fit and went to the gym several times a week. He was married with two children aged 12 and 14 and was highly irritable often flaring with anger easily.

When Daniel first consulted with me I explained the

effects of his childhood trauma on winding up his stress nervous system. As discussed in this chapter, childhood trauma, such as abuse, parents' divorce or other hardship, activates the stress response for a prolonged period of time leading to increased sensitivity of the stress nervous system. Once the brain is sensitive, the brain produces more stress chemicals for any given stress and this continues to keep the stress nervous system wound up, often for life. The increased stress chemicals activate the part of the brain that keeps us awake, leading to insomnia.

I advised Daniel how to unwind the stress nervous system. As he was already exercising I advised him to change activities or add sauna bathing for 20 minutes three or four times a week for three months. I also advised him to attend a mindfulness course to improve his peace of mind.

In three months Daniel noticed he was sleeping better. He was taking only 30 minutes to fall asleep and woke less often during the night. He was now sleeping for seven to eight hours. Over the next few months his energy also spiked and he no longer napped in his van during the day. Eventually he fell asleep within five to ten minutes of going to bed. As a bonus he also felt more relaxed and was less irritable when communicating with his family. For more than a decade now I have advised people to attend the sauna for insomnia, anxiety and depression.

Many people, including myself, have benefited.

The dose of sauna bathing required is 20 minutes three to four times a week for two to three months to unwind the stress nervous system. People always ask about a hot bath or spa pool. Is it as good as the sauna? I usually respond the hotter the better. However, a soak in a hot bath or spa for 20 minutes an hour before you go to sleep can be helpful, especially if you do not have the time or a sauna facility close to home.

A common fact most people do not realise is that sustained levels of concentration can increase the activity of the stress nervous system. This is one factor that may explain stress related symptoms among students, especially around exam time. Cindy, an 18 year old university student, started experiencing sleep disturbance during her mid-year exams. She took longer to get to sleep and often woke during the middle of the night and had difficulty returning to sleep. Even after her exams finished her sleep remained erratic.

During the second half of the year as exams approached her insomnia worsened. She was having trouble falling asleep. Some nights she was awake all night. All she could think about was how desperately she wanted to fall asleep. The worry of not getting a good nights' sleep, tiredness, difficulty concentrating to study and exam pressure all combined to send Cindy into a panic. After the exams she returned home with ongoing insomnia. She tried sedating antihistamines, zopiclone, temazepam and diazepam (Valium). Sometimes these helped for the odd night of okay sleep but her sleep pattern did not return.

Cindy came to see me with her mother, both very distressed. Cindy was on break from university and had enjoyed attending the sauna in the past so I advised her to attend the sauna for 20 minutes every day for a month. Over this period her sleep improved steadily to where she was sleeping eight hours per night without waking in the middle of the night. She stopped taking sleeping tablets and started exercising and reduced her sauna bathing to three times a week.

High levels of concentration increase stress chemicals in the brain and combining exam stress with long hours of concentration late into the night is a potent recipe for disturbing sleep. This is made worse by students giving less priority to exercise and relaxation that protects them from sleep disturbance. I now advise students to stop studying and relax a couple of hours prior to sleeping, otherwise falling asleep may be very difficult. As well as this, putting time aside to exercise or relax is vital as exams loom to remain in good mental and physical health.

CHAPTER 23

YOGA, THE ANCIENT INDIAN REMEDY

Yoga originates from ancient India and is a combination of postures, breathing exercises and meditation. In recent decades yoga has also been taught in heated rooms and called hot yoga. Medical professionals have researched the effects of yoga and found yoga calms the stress nervous system.[111,112] Research carried out at Patanjali Research Foundation, Haridwar, Uttarakhand in India showed regular yoga reduced the activity of the stress nervous system. Participants were taught yoga and were advised to practise at home daily for three months. They were also able to attend one class per week.[109]

Researchers at NKP Salve Institute of Medical Sciences and Research Centre, Maharashtra, India compared the effects of yoga and swimming on the activity of the stress nervous system.[114] One hundred people who did not exercise regularly were separated into two groups that either went swimming or performed yoga for one hour, six days a week. Both swimming and yoga reduced the activity of the stress nervous system as well as reduced blood pressure and pulse rate after three months. Yoga is likely to be as effective as aerobic exercise in influencing the stress nervous system.

Several studies have tested yoga for insomnia, anxiety and depression. One study from Bangalore, India showed 60 minutes of yoga, six days a week for six months improved total sleep time by 60 minutes.[115] This is favourable when compared to common remedies. A review of sleeping tablets showed they improved total sleep time by 41 minutes while cognitive behavioural therapy increased total sleep time by 20 minutes.[116]

Trials of yoga for eight to 12 weeks have shown reductions in anxiety scores. One trial compared yoga five times a week for 12 weeks to the drug diazepam (Valium) for anxiety and found yoga to be more effective than Valium.[117] Another study found twice weekly yoga classes of 90 minutes duration for eight weeks reduced anxiety.[118] Research has shown performing yoga for 45 minutes per day for eight weeks at home after being taught postures reduced anxiety levels in young women.[119]

A yoga breathing class of 45 minutes duration – Sundarshan Kriya Yoga (Sky yoga) – has been developed incorporating slow breathing, rapid breathing and cyclical breathing. A three month trial for people with moderate depression showed significant improvements in 76 percent of people performing Sky yoga.[120] Another study compared four weeks of Sky yoga to an antidepressant and found 70 percent of each group improved significantly.[121]

Shavasana relaxation and breathing for 30 minutes for 30 days was tested by researchers at Punjabi University, India. They found 16 of 25 people in the Shavasana relaxation group were no longer depressed at 30 days compared to 2 out of 25 people in the control group.[122] This is a very short intervention period and two to three months is likely to have a higher response rate.

A trial of yoga and self-hypnosis was performed at Stanford University on people who experienced depression for more than two years.[123] The meditation/yoga included instruction and group practice in meditation, hatha yoga, breathing techniques, guided breathing imagery and mantra repetition. Participants were also taught the meditative practice of surrender – observing thoughts and feelings as they arise and then consciously letting go of these thoughts and feelings using breathing and visualisation techniques. They attended a one-hour class weekly for eight weeks, two workshops of four hours and were asked to practise at home for 30 minutes per day. At the nine month follow-up 77 percent of the group were no longer depressed.

Laughter yoga is a combination of laughter without reason and yogic breathing. A study compared ten sessions of exercise to laughter yoga for depression.[124] Both exercise and laughter yoga showed improvements in depression showing laughter yoga may be a promising intervention for depression. The act of laughing is likely to feed back to the brain to let the brain know that everything is okay and to stop producing stress chemicals.

The studies of yoga as an intervention for insomnia, anxiety and depression need an overhaul. Studies should have a minimum of 45 minutes duration, four sessions per week and be run for a minimum of 12 weeks to ensure an adequate dose is used to reduce the activity of the stress nervous system. The studies performed, however, show the benefit of regular yoga that appeals to some people as a lifestyle choice to remain physically and mentally well.

This chapter has explained that yoga has benefits on mental health. From the previous chapter on sauna, heat also has benefits on mental health. Hot yoga studios have become more popular over the past decade and take advantage of the benefits of heat and yoga. I did hot yoga four to five times a week for a year and taught yoga in a hot room over one year. The combination of the breathing and postures in the heat increases the relaxation potential of yoga. The heat also improves the flexibility of the muscles and allows deeper stretching of the muscles to reduce the stiffness that often occurs as we age. If you have not tried it I would recommend it; however, it does not suit everyone, especially those who cannot tolerate the heat.

CHAPTER 24

MINDFULNESS, MEDITATION AND BREATHING

Mindfulness, meditation and breathing training have been given a new lease of life in the last decade in the western world as treatment for a variety of conditions and to reduce stress. Mindfulness courses and meditation centres that incorporate breathing techniques are teaching people to lead a more relaxed life. The medical research shows mindfulness, meditation and slow breathing all calm the stress nervous system.[125,126,127]

The origins of mindfulness are in Buddhism; however, mindfulness has been introduced free of religious, cultural and ideological factors to explore the mind body connection. A definition of mindfulness is the awareness that emerges through paying attention on purpose in the present moment and non-judgementally to the unfolding of experience moment by moment.[128]

A mindfulness-based stress reduction programme consists of regular group classes to learn facets of mindfulness, meditation (breath focus, body scan and open monitoring) as well as daily home practice. Retreats ranging from a weekend to three months are also available and the research shows these can increase mindfulness and reduce stress with benefits lasting six months after a 10-day course.[129,130,131]

Mindfulness-based programmes are available at schools, hospitals, workplaces, prisons, health centres and churches. Some courses are an hour a week for several weeks, while others are retreats of variable lengths of time. Mindfulness is not achieved after attending one course but requires the implementation of what is learned. Mindfulness is about the process of developing habits over time rather than a definite end goal and is a journey over months, years or decades. Mindfulness increases with time and practice but requires an ongoing commitment. Mindfulness is not about the outcome or fixing anything.

A significant theme in mindfulness is staying in the present moment as this prevents a person worrying about events that have happened in the past that cannot be changed. Staying in the present moment also stops a person worrying about future negative events that may never eventuate. Thus staying in the moment regardless of the activity you are performing, such as washing dishes, gardening, cooking or reading, calms the stress nervous system.

Mindfulness incorporates non-judgement. Without knowing it we often observe something, analyse it and our mind judges what we are observing without even thinking about it. In open monitoring meditation you concentrate on your thoughts and feelings and observe them, almost as if watching your mind as an observer. Often you can look at what thoughts bring about changes in emotions, what creates happiness and what creates sadness. Once you become aware of the voice in the mind that provides judgements, worries and self-criticisms eventually the chatter will subside and leave a sense of stillness and peace. This is the basis of open monitoring meditation and is sometimes referred to as Zen meditation.

Meditation calms the brain, resulting in reduced electrical activity in the brain. Several types of meditation have been investigated to see their effect on the stress nervous system. The National Chiao Tung University in Taiwan, Republic of China compared people who regularly meditated with people who did not meditate and found the activity of the stress nervous system was lower in people who performed regular meditation.[132]

Several brain scans were performed on a Tibetan monk to reveal his mental activity during various meditation practices.[128] The brain scans showed a stable pattern of brain activity during various meditations that have never been seen in the western population. Brain activity patterns were changed at will by the monk when performing different meditation practices such as compassion and devotion. The brain can be controlled by your thoughts and meditation can strongly influence your brain activity.

Researchers at the Department of Medicine, Cedars-Sinai Research Institute studied the effect of transcendental meditation on participants where one group performed meditation while another group received health education for 16 weeks.[127] The activity of the stress nervous system reduced in the group performing transcendental meditation. Meanwhile another study conducted at the Faculty of Medical Sciences, University of Fukui in Japan found Zen meditation can change brain waves and calm the stress nervous system.[133]

In body scan meditation you are aware of different regions of your body and allow yourself to experience how each part feels without trying to change anything. This meditation is often performed lying down and you may start with your big toe and work through the body to the head and then concentrate on the body as a whole. This form of meditation is about getting in touch with the body and at the same time letting go of feelings of needing to get things done.

When faced with danger such as a tiger stalking you, you breathe faster as adrenaline is released throughout the body. Breathing slowly actually sends a signal back to the brain that there is no danger and the parts of the brain producing stress chemicals can relax. Different rates of breathing have been tested and breathing between four and six times per minute has been shown to calm the activity of the stress nervous system. The slow breathing in the disciplines of meditation, yoga, Tai Chi, and Zen meditation is a significant factor in why they create a significant relaxation effect.

A study conducted in Malaysia taught one group to breathe slowly at around six times a minute.[134] They were advised to use this breathing technique at home for five minutes, four times a day and whenever feeling stressed. One week after the training finished anxiety and depression levels reduced in the breathing group. In San Diego, California researchers at the California School of Professional Psychology at Alliant International University compared two groups of 30 people. One group was taught relaxation abdominal breathing at classes they attended once a week for 45 minutes for six weeks and encouraged to practise breathing for 20 minutes per day. The group performing deep breathing had measurable reductions in the activity of the stress nervous system at follow-up three months after classes finished.[126]

Researchers at Harvard Medical School in Boston looked into the activity of the stress nervous system with breathing used in yoga and meditation.[135] They found slow relaxed breathing reduced the activity of the stress nervous system.

Recently I have been practising deep breathing for 20 minutes using a monitor that measures the stress nervous system activity and found after around five minutes my stress nervous system activity starts to reduce. Slow breathing is an excellent technique to calm the stress nervous system as there is no equipment required and no cost. Slow breathing will effectively unwind the stress nervous system over three to four months and improve stress related conditions when performed daily.

To practise deep breathing find a comfortable place to sit or lie down, concentrate on your normal breaths and then take a few deep breaths slowly that expand your abdomen fully. The breath can come in through the mouth or nose, depending on what feels right for you. It feels as if the air coming in goes deep into your lower belly. Alternate several deep and normal breaths. Shallow breathing normally feels constricted and tense while deep breathing often feels relaxing. Once you are warmed up you can practise deep breathing with your hand on the abdomen. As you breathe in your abdomen rises and as you breathe out your abdomen should fall. You can count to five as you breathe in and count to five as you breathe out.

Meditation is likely to be an essential part of improving stress related symptoms in the long term. In the last few months of researching this book I came across articles that found reduced GABA levels in the brain in patients with depression,[22] panic attacks,[23] and insomnia.[24] GABA neurones make up 20 percent of the brain and act to dampen electricity in most parts of the brain. As stress chemicals are the on switch to many parts of the brain and create electricity leading to symptoms of insomnia, anxiety, depression and irritability, GABA is the off switch. GABA dampens electricity. Unfortunately, the prolonged release of stress chemicals that occurs with long term stress, such as childhood trauma, both winds up the stress nervous system and reduces GABA levels in the brain

A few trials of meditation have measured GABA levels in the brain. Researchers at York University in Toronto Canada compared two groups.[136] One group performed meditation for one hour while the other group watched television for one hour. The GABA levels increased in the brain only in the meditation group. A trial conducted at University of California, Irvine compared the effects of one hour of meditation and one hour of reading.[137] They found only meditation increased GABA levels.

My suspicion is that meditation reduces the electricity in the brain more than reading or watching television that still require some parts of the brain to be electrically active. The more often the electricity in the brain is reduced to low levels by meditation the more likely the GABA neurones are to produce GABA. Prior to this information, I was meditating for 20 minutes but now have increased this to 60 minutes per day in the hope of restoring GABA levels over three to four months. This may help stress related symptoms in the longer term. After decades of disturbed sleep, from time to time I suspect restoring the GABA levels in the brain may lead to fewer relapses of sleep disturbance for myself.

Mindfulness based stress reduction has been compared to sleeping tablets in a trial conducted at the University of Minnesota, Minneapolis and found to be as effective as sleeping tablets in improving sleep after eight weeks and at the five month follow-up.[138] Meditation was performed for 45 minutes per day for eight weeks followed by 20 minutes daily. At the five month follow-up total sleep time had improved by 34 minutes from six hours 31 minutes to seven hours and five minutes in the mindfulness based stress reduction group.

Researchers at Rush University in Chicago developed a mindfulness-based programme developed for insomnia including breathing and meditation and tested this therapy for people with insomnia.[139] Participants were advised to perform mindfulness meditation for 30 to 45 minutes at least six days a week and to keep a meditation and sleep diary. At three months 71 percent experienced improved sleep and at six months 76 percent of participants were sleeping better. The total sleep time of participants increased by 40 minutes.

Several trials have looked at mindfulness-based cognitive therapy to reduce the recurrence of depression. Overall it reduced the recurrence of depression by 35 percent when averaged over several studies. Two of the studies found it was at least as effective as antidepressant medication.[136,137] A group of researchers in the United Kingdom where the lead researcher worked out of the University of Exeter, Devon compared mindfulness-based cognitive therapy to antidepressants for relapse of depression. They found over 15 months, 47 percent of people relapsed into depression in the mindfulness group compared to 60 percent in the antidepressant group. The study also found 75 percent of patients in the mindfulness group completely stopped using antidepressant medication.[141]

Mindfulness, meditation and breathing are useful tools in today's society that lead to long term improvement of insomnia, anxiety and depression. These tools also allow people to live a more balanced life.

CHAPTER 25

TAI CHI – YIN AND YANG

Tai Chi is an ancient form of exercise in oriental cultures to enhance balance and body awareness. The term refers to a philosophy of the forces of yin and yang. Tai Chi is based on softness and awareness instead of force and resistance and combines movement with breathing. Tai Chi has been shown to reduce the activity of the stress nervous system after a 40 minute session.[142] The same study found the activity of the stress nervous system was lower in people who regularly performed Tai Chi. A trial was conducted at National Yang-Ming University School of Medicine, Taipei, Taiwan where people were randomised from the general population to perform Tai Chi for 40 minutes seven days a week for three months.[143] The stress nervous system activity reduced significantly in the Tai Chi group and showed no changes in the group who did not perform Tai Chi.

Several randomised control trials of Tai Chi have found it improves sleep. At the University of California, Los Angeles researchers randomised 112 people to attend Tai Chi 40 minutes three times a week or attend a health education programme for 16 weeks.[144] After 16 weeks the time to get to sleep improved 31 percent and sleep duration improved 19 percent in the Tai Chi group. Both sleep measures improved twice as much in the Tai Chi group compared to the health education group.

The Oregon Research Institute at Willamette University, Salem, Oregon conducted a study of the effects of three 60 minute sessions per week over 24 weeks on sleep.[145] They randomised 118 people to either Tai Chi or low impact exercise. They found Tai Chi was effective in improving several sleep measures. Total sleep time increased by 48 minutes and daytime sleepiness also improved.

The Institute of Gerontology, Heidelberg University, Heidelberg, Germany studied the effects of attending Tai Chi 60 minutes twice a week for six months on sleep quality.[146] The study employed the Pittsburgh sleep quality index to measure sleep quality with a score of over five representing poor sleep. Only the Tai Chi group showed significant improvements in sleep with the initial average score being nine and the final score being less than four.

Tai Chi has also been studied as an intervention for anxiety and depression. At Taipei Medical University, Taiwan, China a randomised control trial of Tai Chi, three times a week for 12 weeks (10 minute warm-up, 30 minutes Tai Chi and 10 minutes warm-down) showed significant reductions in anxiety scores.[147] They estimated Tai Chi elevated heart rate to around

60 percent of a person's maximum heart rate creating a significant aerobic exercise effect.

A study of Tai Chi performed at the Hong Kong University in Hong Kong, Republic of China investigated the effects of three 45 minute sessions of Tai Chi per week for three months.[148] The Tai Chi group reduced their depression scores 52 percent while the control group increased their depression scores. A review of Tai Chi for depression found Tai Chi had positive outcomes in several randomised control trials.[149.]

CHAPTER 26

HOW DOES MEDICATION WORK?

Medications attach to receptors and change electricity in different parts of the brain. Changing electricity in the reticular formation may change sleep while changing electricity in the amygdala may change anxiety and panic attacks. Changing several sites of the brain, including the hypothalamus, may alter depression. Medications for insomnia, anxiety and depression have significant overlap and many target stress chemicals such as noradrenaline, serotonin, adrenaline and dopamine receptors.

In the 1950s the first antidepressant iproniazid, originally developed for tuberculosis, was found to increase serotonin in the brain. In the early trials of iproniazid for tuberculosis, researchers observed that people showed greater vitality and increased social activity.[150] There were even reports of patients dancing and partying in the tuberculosis wards. Reports started appearing of the mood enhancing effects of this drug and the term antidepressant was coined in this era. One year later 400,000 people were taking it for depression. After this period several other drugs were developed for depression.

Ideally, medications for insomnia, anxiety and

depression should unwind the stress nervous system for long term effectiveness. Unfortunately, studies have shown the opposite; antidepressants, such as tricyclic antidepressants (amitriptyline and nortriptyline) and serotonin reuptake inhibitors (SSRIs) such as fluoxetine, increase the activity of the stress nervous system.[151]

Antidepressants that increase activity of the stress nervous system may increase insomnia, anxiety and depression for patients if taken long term. Researchers from Amsterdam performed more than 20,000 measurements over 20 years on more than 11,000 people. They compared measurements when people were either taking or not taking antidepressants. They found tricyclic antidepressants increased activity of the stress nervous system.[152] Many medications that are designed to help stress related conditions may help in the short term but may lose effectiveness as they wind up the stress nervous system.

The effect of venlafaxine and mirtazapine on the activity of the stress nervous system was tested in patients with depression.[153] Measures were taken after stopping medication for a week and then after 14 and 28 days of treatment. Depressed patients had increased activity of the stress nervous system after taking venlafaxine or mirtazapine. The study stated that clinicians should consider the effect of antidepressants on the activity of the stress nervous system when selecting antidepressants as those that increase stress nervous system activity are likely to increase the future risk of developing depression.

Medications increasing stress nervous system activity have been found to cause early death. The risk of early death was 30 to 60 percent higher for post-menopausal women taking antidepressants when compared to those not taking antidepressants.[154] Antipsychotics, including chlorpromazine, clozapine, olanzapine, quetiapine, haloperidol, flupenthixol, sulpiride, amisulpiride, aripiprazole and risperidone, also increase stress nervous system activity.[155]

CHAPTER 27

MEDICATION FOR INSOMNIA

Low dose antidepressants and hypnotics, such as temazepam, are often prescribed to treat insomnia. In 2015, 5.3 million scripts of low dose antidepressants and 3.4 million scripts of hypnotics were prescribed for insomnia in the United States.[156]

Sleeping tablets work by reducing electricity in the parts of the brain that keep you awake. There are, however, a great variety of medications that create sedation and may help sleep such as antihistamines, antipsychotics, antidepressants and anti-epileptic medication. These tablets act on a variety of brain receptors including Gamma aminobutyric acid (GABA), histamine, serotonin, acetylcholine, noradrenaline and adrenaline receptors.

The two most commonly prescribed sleeping tablets are benzodiazepines and antidepressants. Benzodoazepines, (diazepam and temazepam) on average reduce the time to get to sleep by 15 minutes and increase total sleep time by 41 minutes in people with acute insomnia. Antidepressants reduce the time to get to sleep on average by 12 minutes.[157]

Unfortunately, antidepressants such as amitriptyline are not specific for one part of the brain and act on several parts of the brain creating side effects. Side effects include dry mouth, difficulty urinating, constipation, fine tremor, drowsiness and weight gain as well as reduced memory and concentration. With low dose antidepressants 25 percent of people develop headache, 20 percent experience dizziness, 20 percent of people gain weight and 70 percent develop dry mouth.

Many tablets can disturb sleep as they act on receptors that increase electricity in the sleep centres. Fluoxetine, an antidepressant, disturbs sleep, increasing the time taken to get to sleep and reducing total sleep duration. Fluoxetine also suppresses REM sleep. Up to 20 percent of patients taking these tablets experience worsening of insomnia.

Melatonin is a hormone produced in the brain that has low levels in the daytime and increased levels at night time. Many studies have been performed for melatonin tablets for insomnia and on the whole some studies show some benefit, while many show no benefit.

Treatment of insomnia may require using all the tools in the toolbox including medications for the short term while starting regular exercise, sauna, yoga, Tai Chi or meditation, depending on your preference. If sleep is improved, this will often help symptoms of anxiety and depression. Often tablets are a personal preference and a trial and error approach is often required to find a tablet that works without too many unwanted effects.

All the variety of tablets mentioned earlier, such as antidepressants, antihistamines, antipsychotics or antiepileptics, can be taken in small doses. These types of sedating medications are not usually addictive and can be taken for weeks to months while people develop lifestyle habits that will naturally help people sleep. As people are different a trial and error approach is often required before a suitable tablet that improves sleep without too many side effects can be found.

Sleeping tablets such as benzodiazepines (diazepam, temazepam or zopiclone) may be used once or twice a week to help sleep. Taken this way, tolerance (where the tablet stops working) and addiction are less likely to occur.

CHAPTER 28

MEDICATION FOR ANXIETY

A variety of medications, including benzodiazepines, beta blockers and antidepressants, are used to treat anxiety. Tricyclic antidepressants (amitriptyline, nortriptyline) and newer antidepressants, such as serotonin and noradrenaline reuptake inhibitors, are prescribed for anxiety.

Anxiety disorder is commonly treated with benzodiazepines (alprazolam, diazepam, lorazepam and clonazepam). Benzodiazepines are highly addictive and people develop tolerance whereby the medication stops working and higher doses are required. Despite the use of daily benzodiazepines for more than a year most people still had residual symptoms of anxiety while taking tablets. When they stopped the tablets they experienced withdrawal symptoms.[159] If people managed to go five weeks without tablets their anxiety was better than when they were taking benzodiazepines.

A study of more than 4,000 people who were regularly prescribed benzodiazepines from their general practitioner found more than 75 percent were extremely unwell with 60 percent of patients experiencing anxiety and 60 percent experiencing depression.[160] Benzodiazepines are not recommended for long term treatment due to addiction and tolerance (where a tablet stops working and increased doses are required) developing. Drugs such as paroxetine and venlafaxine are usually preferred over benzodiazepines for the treatment of anxiety disorders.

Most studies show that 10 to 20 percent more people respond to antidepressants for anxiety than placebo tablets.[161] At three months venlafaxine helped 58 percent of patients with social anxiety disorder versus 33 percent responding to placebo tablets.[162] In another study at six months venlafaxine helped 69 percent of patients with social anxiety disorder versus up to 46 percent improvement with placebo tablets.[163] Paroxetine and escitalopram have also shown similar improvements for anxiety disorder.

Propanolol has been found to be as effective as benzodiazepines for panic attacks.[164] It has been used for performance anxiety in musicians, people taking exams, stage fright and for surgeons performing operations. Propanolol suppresses many of the physical symptoms of panic attack, such as palpitations and racing heart, by directly blocking adrenaline receptors throughout the body.

CHAPTER 29

ANTIDEPRESSANT MEDICATION

There are many different antidepressants on the market including the older generation tricyclic antidepressants (amitriptyline, nortriptyline) and newer antidepressants selective serotonin reuptake inhibitors (SSRI), serotonin-noradrenaline reuptake inhibitors (SNRI) and monoamine oxidase inhibitors to name a few. Ideally, antidepressants should unwind the stress nervous system for long term effectiveness. Antidepressants wind up the stress nervous system and tend to lose their effectiveness for many after six months. Despite antidepressants being the number one prescribed treatment for depression, inactive placebo tablets produce at least 75 percent of the effect of antidepressant tablets.[165]

Fluoxetine (Prozac) is the most common antidepressant prescribed. Common side effects include agitation, changes in sexual function, erectile dysfunction, failure to orgasm, dizziness, dry mouth, headache, psychological and emotion changes such as blunted emotions or aggression and weight gain.

In adolescents who are depressed, three times as many who were taking antidepressants committed suicide compared to those not taking antidepressants.[166]

As antidepressants wind up the stress nervous system a percentage of individuals probably become more depressed. This may be one reason for the increased rates of suicide in adolescents in people taking antidepressants.

A study investigating mindfulness-based stress reduction to prevent relapses of depression gives some insight into the effectiveness of antidepressants in the long term.[167] Firstly different antidepressants were prescribed to improve depression. Initially, sertraline was prescribed and if there was no effect mirtazapine was prescribed. Fifty two percent of people taking antidepressants improved. After seven months half the study group continued antidepressants and the other half underwent mindfulness-based cognitive therapy to see who would relapse back into depression. Thirty eight percent of the mindfulness group became depressed and 46 percent of the antidepressant group became depressed.

This study shows antidepressants are not working long term in the majority of patients. Out of 100 people initially taking antidepressants 52 went into remission. At 18 months only 24 people remained without depression. In the short-term antidepressants work; however, in the longer term they do not work as well as sauna, Tai Chi, yoga, meditation and exercise as these activities unwind the stress nervous system. Research shows therapies aimed at reducing the activity of the stress nervous system have greater effectiveness than antidepressants in the long term.

Novel Medications for Depression

In my review of the medical literature while researching this book I stumbled across some novel agents that seem to be helpful in improving depression. Ketamine has been found to have a profound and quick effect on major depression that has not responded to usual treatment. It is given by intravenous infusion in hospitals. One study of people with major depression that tested intravenous infusion of ketamine versus placebo showed 71 percent responded at one day and 35 percent at one week.[168] No patients in the placebo infusion group responded at one or seven days.

Another trial of ketamine infusion has confirmed an antidepressant activity and showed 71 percent responded compared to six percent of patients given placebo infusion.[169] This rapid improvement in depression is important especially for acutely suicidal patients as most antidepressants will take several weeks to take effect.

Nitrous oxide, otherwise known as laughing gas, has been studied for treatment resistant major depression.[170] Patients that had failed at least three different antidepressant tablets were included in this trial of nitrous oxide gas versus placebo gas. Patients received 50 percent nitrous oxide/50 percent oxygen versus 50 percent nitrogen/50 percent oxygen by inhalation for one hour for two sessions one week apart. At 24 hours

35 percent of patients responded to nitrous oxide gas.

Antidepressants are reasonably effective in the first six months with approximately 65 percent responding and they may be a useful tool to boost mood while people start regular exercise, sauna, meditation/breathing, yoga or Tai Chi to reduce the activity of the stress nervous system. After three to four months these therapies should have started to improve mood and a decision can be made to reduce antidepressants slowly if mood has improved. Ideally, people should develop lifelong habits to maintain physical and mental health and prevent symptoms relapsing.

CHAPTER 30

COGNITIVE BEHAVIOURAL THERAPY

Cognitive behavioural therapy is a goal oriented therapy to help clients change unhelpful thinking and behaviour patterns. An example is someone who believes the world is a dangerous place and they cannot trust anyone, so they fear leaving the house. Cognitive behavioural therapy would examine the belief that the world is a dangerous place, the emotion of fear that is produced and the behaviour of not leaving the house. Cognitive behavioural therapy often involves a weekly session for around four months to make meaningful change.

A review of 21 trials of patients with insomnia comparing sleeping tablets and cognitive behavioural therapy found sleeping tablets reduced the time to get to sleep by 15 minutes and improved total sleep time by 41 minutes.[116] Cognitive behavioural therapy reduced the time to get to sleep by 17 minutes and increased total sleep time by 20 minutes. The review concluded sleeping tablets and cognitive behavioural therapy were equally effective in the short term with the costs of cognitive behavioural therapy greater than tablets.

Studies show cognitive behavioural therapy is useful

for anxiety disorders including generalised anxiety disorder, social anxiety disorder, panic disorder and post-traumatic stress disorder.[171] A study looking into long term results for anxiety disorders found approximately 50 percent of people who responded to cognitive behavioural therapy maintained their improvement one year after therapy finished.

Cognitive behavioural therapy in most studies is equivalent in effect to antidepressants. Over 100 studies have investigated the effectiveness of cognitive behavioural therapy. The National Institute of Mental Health Treatment of Depression Collaborative Research Program in the United States performed a trial of around 250 people in multiple study centres and its results are representative of most of these studies. They found cognitive behavioural therapy and antidepressants gave similar results. In the cognitive behavioural therapy group around 50 percent were no longer depressed after 16 to 20 sessions over 16 weeks.[172] In this study a similar number were no longer depressed after taking antidepressants. Another trial comparing antidepressant medication, cognitive behavioural therapy and placebo for eight weeks found cognitive behavioural therapy had a similar effect to placebo tablets at eight weeks.[173] This study shows more than eight weeks are required for cognitive behavioural therapy to improve depression.

When cognitive behavioural therapy is on offer,

the major factor is patient preference between cognitive behavioural therapy and antidepressants. Some patients prefer cognitive behavioural therapy while others may prefer a pill. Cognitive behavioural therapy has been historically carried out one on one with a counsellor or psychologist which can create cost barriers for many people. There are, however, group sessions and increasingly online versions are now available. Acceptance and Commitment Therapy (ACT) and Focussed Acceptance and Commitment Therapy (FACT) are relative newcomers that have sprouted from cognitive behavioural therapy and offer much shorter and more cost effective therapy than cognitive behavioural therapy with similar outcomes in the medical literature for insomnia, anxiety and depression.

CONCLUSION

Everyone has experienced poor sleep, moments of anxiety and sadness. These feelings are part of being human as much as it is to feel joy and happiness. Some might say unless you have experienced sadness you may not realise what true joy and happiness feel like. When poor sleep, anxiety and depression take over your life, robbing you of your vitality and energy, you can take a downward spiral. You can experience poor confidence, reduced self-esteem, lose your job and relationships can suffer. Sometimes people can take their own lives resulting in devastation for family and friends. In New Zealand almost weekly you hear of a friend or acquaintance who knows someone who has taken their own life.

In a world that is evolving rapidly we are fast forgetting that we are animals who, due to our ability to codify knowledge (read and write), have passed on knowledge to future generations to advance technology, speed up the pace of life and dominate all species that dwell on earth. Our minds and bodies have not kept pace and have not had a chance to catch up to the requirements of sedentary living, an unlimited food supply and a vast array of technological and luxury goods that we aspire to own.

Your mind and body are the most important

commodities you have in the world. You need time to look after your mind and body. You need to spend each moment as if it is sand passing through the hourglass, never to return. As sand cannot reverse against gravity, time ticks away each second, minute, hour, day, month and year. What you do each day will determine the state of your mind and body in years and decades to come. This will determine how you feel, your health, vitality, energy, sleep and mood. There are no quick cures, easy remedies, vitamins, minerals, drugs or diet that will cure your insomnia, anxiety or depression. The reason these are touted is for profit, as the cause of these conditions has been elusive.

After spending many years looking at these problems I have tested the strategies in this book with countless patients who remind me of how well they feel after many years of poor health. It has been a pleasure seeing people turn their lives around. I always say to them I cannot cure you but only guide you to help yourself once you understand your condition.

When I started the book I looked at insomnia, anxiety and depression as stress related symptoms and, like 99 percent of doctors, believed people who experienced these disorders were structurally similar to the rest of the population. After looking at the research it seems people with prolonged stress are different. Not only is the stress nervous system significantly more sensitive but parts of the brain and body involved in the stress response grow. The adrenal gland is 70 percent larger and the pituitary gland 30 percent larger in people experiencing depression. The brain also has significant differences with reductions in grey matter volume including parts of the brain important for memory and concentration (hippocampus). Furthermore, the 20 percent of the brain that is responsible for reducing electricity in the brain (GABA neurons) also shrink. Fortunately, for all the people suffering around the world, all these changes are reversible.

Examining psychological beliefs and increasing social interaction to reduce loneliness are also important in the long-term rehabilitation of patients with insomnia, anxiety and depression. This is going to be a lot easier if changes to the stress pathways and brain are restored back to normal. People will be able to process past trauma, examine faulty beliefs and interact with people more easily with a calm mind. Developing habits that calm the stress nervous system and following this up with a stint of meditation to grow the neurones that reduce electricity in the brain, may prevent relapses of insomnia, anxiety and depression in individuals. This may be a game changer as these symptoms often plague someone for most of their lives and follow a recurrent pattern.

We need to use all the tools in the toolbox to solve

our mental health problems. This includes the judicious use of medication. Taking antidepressants, sleeping tablets or medication for anxiety can be useful for many, especially in the short term. If patients respond to medications this may increase their motivation to incorporate habits into their lives that will unwind their stress nervous system. Over decades I have maintained an exercise habit for around half an hour five times a week as well as walking for recreation and attending sauna/spa facilities. More recently, since learning about the benefits of meditation for the brain, I have also added at least 20 minutes of meditation daily to my habits. Having experienced regular nightmares and night sweats for decades, these are the habits that are eliminating sleep disturbance. Now my sleep is disturbed very rarely and the nightmares have also subsided. I have encouraged my children to exercise regularly, leading by example and ensuring they have memberships to a gym to ensure they have the facilities to maintain the habits that will ensure sound mental health and wellbeing.

Once people start on their journey, it is a lifelong habit that will turn their lives around and result in a good night's sleep where you wake like a box of birds with boundless energy and experience a deep joy that is not robbed quickly by day to day events. Improving the quality of someone's life for what may be several decades of life is the most pleasing part of my job and research. I hope this book helps you gain an understanding of your condition and conviction to develop habits to improve the quality of your life for decades to come.

Index

ACKNOWLEDGEMENTS

My thanks go out to all the patients who have allowed their stories to appear in this book. All names have been changed so patients can remain anonymous. Thanks to my wife for her support while writing this book. The four year journey to write this book certainly was not possible without her support. Thanks to my children, mother and family for their support.

Thanks to Sathna Kanji, Lisa Smith, Jessica Kanji, Ashwin Patel, Keelan Kanji, Ataya Kanji and all the other people who proof read the book and gave ideas on improvement. A special thanks to Linda Cassells, Janene Bone, Nitha Palakshappa, Sophie Ball, Sarah Hood, Tara Satyanand, Gareth Eyres and Stephen Buetow for editing and proofreading the manuscript. Thanks to Sam Cawthorn for advice on the cover and to Luke Williamson from Halcyon design for producing the cover. My thanks also to Bruce Arroll, John Windsor, Rachel Page and Anil Thapliyal for endorsements and Chris Bullen for writing the foreword.

This book has been rewritten several times and what started as a fully illustrated book has finished being a short book that is hopefully readable to the layperson but also may serve as a reference tool for health professionals who look after people experiencing insomnia, anxiety and depression.

Dr Giresh Kanji

April 2019

REFERENCES

1. Murray Stein et al. "Impairment associated with sleep problems in the community: relationship to physical and mental health comorbidity." Psychosomatic Medicine 70 (2008): 913–919.
2. Dugal Campbel et al. "Characteristics of a conditioned response in human subjects during extinction trials following a single traumatic conditioning trial." J Abnorm Psychol. 68 (1964): 629-639.
3. Benedetto Farina et al. "Heart rate and heart rate variability modification in chronic insomnia." Patients Behavioral Sleep Medicine 12 (2014): 290–306.
4. Andre Pittig et al. "Heart rate and heart rate variability in panic, social anxiety, obsessive–compulsive, and generalized anxiety disorders at baseline and in response to relaxation and hyperventilation." International Journal of Psychophysiology 87, 1 (2013): 19-27.
5. Andre Brunoni. "Heart rate variability is a trait marker of major depressive disorder: evidence from the sertraline vs. electric current therapy to treat depression clinical study." International Journal of Neuropsychopharmacology 16 (2013): 1937–1949.
6. Julian Montaquila et al. "Heart rate variability and vagal tone in schizophrenia: a review." Journal of Psychiatric Research 69 (2015): 57–66.
7. Marcus Agelink et al. "Relationship between major depression and heart rate variability. Clinical consequences and implications for antidepressive treatment." Psychiatry Research 113, 1–2 (2002): 139–49.
8. Marcus Agelink et al. "Improvement of neurocardial vagal dysfunction after successful antidepressive treatment with electro-convulsive therapy." European Psychiatry 13, S4 (1998): 259.
9. Irfan Barutcu et al. "Cigarette smoking and heart rate variability: dynamic influence of parasympathetic and sympathetic manoeuvres." Annals of Noninvasive Electrocardiology 10, 3 (2005): 324–29.
10. Christopher Harte et al. "Association between smoking and heart rate variability among individuals with depression." Annals of Behavioral Medicine 46, 1 (2013): 73–80.
11. Pekka Koskinen et al. "Acute alcohol intake decreases short-term heart rate variability in healthy subjects." Clinical Science 87, 2 (1994): 225–30.
12. Paulo Bau et al. "Acute ingestion of alcohol and cardiac autonomic modulation in healthy volunteers." Alcohol 45, 2 (2011): 123–29.
13. Jonas Spaak et al. "Dose-related effects of red wine and alcohol on heart rate variability." American Journal of Physiology – Heart and Circulatory Physiology 298, 6 (2010): 2226–31.

14. Richard Famularo et al. "Psychiatric diagnoses of maltreated children: preliminary findings." Journal of the American Academy of Child & Adolescent Psychiatry 31, 5 (1992): 863–67.
15. Kenneth Kendler et al. "Childhood parental loss and adult psychopathology in women. a twin study perspective." Archives of General Psychiatry 49, 2 (1992): 109–16.
16. C. Heim and C. Nemeroff. "The role of childhood trauma in the neurobiology of mood and anxiety disorders: preclinical and clinical studies." Biological Psychiatry 49, 12 (2001): 1023–39.
17. Vincent Felitti et al. "Relationship of childhood abuse and household dysfunction to many of the leading causes of death in adults." American Journal of Preventive Medicine 14, 4 (1998): 245–58.
18. Akinori Masuda et al. "Intra- and extra-familial adverse childhood experiences and a history of childhood psychosomatic disorders among Japanese university students." BioPsychoSocial Medicine 1 (2007): 1-9.
19. Tiffany Field et al. "Prenatal depression effects on the fetus and the newborn." Infant Behavior and Development 27, 2 (2004): 216–29.
20. Brenda Lundy et al. "Prenatal depression effects on neonates." Infant Behavior and Development 22, 1 (1999): 119–29.
21. Setsuko Sahara. "The fraction of cortical GABAergic neurons is constant from near the start of cortical neurogenesis to adulthood." J Neurosci. 32, 14 (2012): 4755–4761.
22. John Winkelman et al. "Reduced brain GABA in primary insomnia: preliminary data from 4T proton magnetic resonance spectroscopy (1H-MRS)." Sleep 31 (2008): 1499-1506.
23. Andrew Goddard et al. "Reductions in occipital cortex GABA levels in panic disorder detected with 1H magnetic resonance spectroscopy." Archives of General Psychiatry. June, 58, 6 (2001): 556-561.
24. Gerard Sanacora et al. "Reduced cortical G-aminobutyric acid levels in depressed patients determined by proton magnetic resonance spectroscopy." Ach Gen Psychiatry 56 (1999): 1043-1047.
25. Erkki Kronholm et al. "Trends in self-reported sleep duration and insomnia-related symptoms in Finland from 1972 to 2005: a comparative review and re-analysis of Finnish population samples." Journal of Sleep Research 17, 1 (2008): 54–62.
26. Charlotte Schoenborn. "Health habits of U.S. adults, 1985: the 'Alameda 7' revisited." Public Health Reports 101, 6 (1986): 571–80.
27. Maria Calem et al. "Increased prevalence of insomnia and changes in hypnotics use in England over 15 years." Sleep 35,3 (2012): 377-84.

28. Sairam Parthasarathy et al. "Persistent insomnia is associated with mortality risk." The American Journal of Medicine 128, 3 (2015): 268–275.

29. Hannah Morphy et al. "Epidemiology of insomnia: a longitudinal study in a UK population." Sleep 30, 3 (2007): 274–80.

30. Charles Morin et al. "The natural history of insomnia: a population-based 3-year longitudinal study." Archives of Internal Medicine 169, 5 (2009): 447–53.

31. Christer Janson et al. "Insomnia in men-a 10-year prospective population based study." Sleep 24, 4 (2001): 425– 30.

32. Catherine Jefferson et al. "Sleep hygiene practices in a population-based sample of insomniacs." Sleep 28, 5 (2005): 611–615.

33. Laura Juliano et al. "Caffeine: pharmacology and clinical effects," in Principles of Addiction Medicine, Third Edition.

34. Writing Group for the Women's Health Initiative Investigators. "Risks and benefits of estrogen plus progestin in healthy postmenopausal women: principal results from the women's health initiative randomized controlled trial." JAMA 288, 3 (2002): 321–33.

35. James Carmody et al. "Mindfulness training for coping with hot flashes: results of a randomized trial." Menopause 18, 6 (2011): 611–20.

36. Rui Afonso et al. "Yoga decreases insomnia in postmenopausal women: a randomized clinical trial." Menopause 19, 2 (2012): 186–93.

37. Denise Oliveira et al. "Effect of massage in postmenopausal women with insomnia – a pilot study." Clinics 66, 2 (2011): 343–46.

38. Barbara Sternfeld et al. "Efficacy of exercise for menopausal symptoms: a randomized controlled trial." Menopause 21, 4 (2014): 330–38.

39. Vered Stearns et al. "Paroxetine controlled release in the treatment of menopausal hot flashes: a randomized controlled trial." JAMA 289, 21 (2003): 2827–34.

40. Vered Stearns et al. "Paroxetine is an effective treatment for hot flashes: results from a prospective randomized clinical trial." Journal of Clinical Oncology 23, 28 (2005): 6919–30.

41. Lee Cohen et al. "Efficacy of omega-3 for vasomotor symptoms treatment: a randomized controlled trial." Menopause 21, 4 (2014): 347–54.

42. Alexandros Vgontzas et al. "Chronic insomnia is associated with nyctohemeral activation of the hypothalamic-pituitary-adrenal axis: clinical implications." The Journal of Clinical Endocrinology & Metabolism 86, 8 (2001): 3787–3794.

43. Katherine Rimes et al. Cortisol output in adolescents with chronic fatigue syndrome: Pilot study on the comparison with healthy adolescents and change after cognitive behavioural guided self-help treatment. Journal of Psychosomatic Research 77 (2014) 409–414.

44. Aaron Laposky et al. "Sleep and circadian rhythms: key components in the regulation of energy metabolism." FEBS Letters, Metabolic Disease 582, 1 (2008): 142–51.

45. Juergen Henning et al. "Changes in cortisol secretion during shiftwork: implications for tolerance to shiftwork?" Ergonomics 41, 5 (1998): 610–21.

46. Vikram Yeragani et al. "Decreased heart rate variability in panic disorder patients: a study of power- spectral analysis of heart rate." Psychiatry Research 46, 1 (1993): 89–103.

47. Bridget Grant et al. "Prevalence, correlates, co-morbidity, and comparative disability of DSM-IV generalized anxiety disorder in the USA: results from the National Epidemiologic Survey on Alcohol and Related Conditions." Psychological Medicine 35 (2005): 1747–1759.

48. Hans-Ulrich Wittchen. "Generalized anxiety disorder: prevalence, burden, and cost to society." Depression and Anxiety 16, 4 (2002): 162–71.

49. M. Stein and D. Stein. "Social anxiety disorder." Lancet 371, 9618 (2008): 1115–25.

50. Ministry of Health. "Patterns of antidepressant drug prescribing and intentional self-harm outcomes in New Zealand: an ecological study." (2007).

51. Mental Health Foundation. "Mental health foundation: quick facts and stats 2014." (2014).

52. T. Bedirhan Üstün and Ron Kessler. "Global burden of depressive disorders: the issue of duration." The British Journal of Psychiatry 181, 3 (2002): 181–83.

53. Jan Spijker et al. "Duration of major depressive episodes in the general population: results from the Netherlands mental health survey and incidence study (NEMESIS)." The British Journal of Psychiatry 181, 3 (2002): 208–13.

54. Hannie Comijs et al. "The two-year course of late- life depression; results from the Netherlands study of depression in older persons." BMC Psychiatry 15 (2015): 15-20.

55. Ronald Kessler et al. "Prevalence, correlates, and course of minor depression and major depression in the national comorbidity survey." Journal of Affective Disorders 45 (1997): 19–30.

56. Madhukar Trivedi et al. "Evaluation of outcomes with citalopram for depression using measurement-based care in STAR*D: implications for clinical practice." The American Journal of Psychiatry 163, 1 (2006): 28–40.

57. Dan Blazer et al. "The prevalence and distribution of major depression in a national community sample: the national comorbidity survey." The American Journal of Psychiatry 151, 7 (1994): 979–86.

58. Jose Luis Ayuso-Mateos et al. "Depressive disorders in Europe: prevalence figures from the ODIN study." The British Journal of Psychiatry 179, 4 (2001): 308–16.

59. Fiona Muir et al. "Depression in medical students: current insights." Advances in Medical Education and Practice 9 (2018): 323-333.

60. Kenneth Kendler et al. "Stressful life events and previous episodes in the etiology of major depression in women: an evaluation of the 'kindling' hypothesis." The American Journal of Psychiatry 157, 8 (2000): 1243–51.

61. Constance Hammen et al. "Depression and sensitization to stressors among young women as a function of childhood adversity." Journal of Consulting and Clinical Psychology 68, 5 (2000): 782–87.

62. Kate Harkness et al. "Gender differences in life events prior to onset of major depressive disorder: the moderating effect of age." Journal of Abnormal Psychology 119, 4 (2010): 791–803.

63. Kenneth Kendler et al. "Life event dimensions of loss, humiliation, entrapment, and danger in the prediction of onsets of major depression and generalized anxiety." Archives of General Psychiatry 60, 8 (2003): 789–96.

64. R. Kessler and E. Bromet. "The epidemiology of depression across cultures." Annual Review of Public Health 34 (2013): 119.

65. Laura Andrade et al. "The epidemiology of major depressive episodes: results from the international consortium of psychiatric epidemiology (ICPE) surveys." International Journal of Methods in Psychiatric Research 12, 1 (2003): 3–21.

66. Robert Carney et al. "Depression, heart rate variability, and acute myocardial infarction." Circulation 104 (2001): 2024-2028.

67. Maria Karavidas et al. "Preliminary results of an open label study of heart rate variability biofeedback for the treatment of major depression." Applied Psychophysiology and Biofeedback 32, 1 (2007): 19–30.

68. Robert Rubin et al. "Adrenal gland volume in major depression. Increase during the depressive episode and decrease with successful treatment." Arch Gen Psychiatry 52, 3 (1995): 213-8.

69. K. Ranga Rama Krishnan et al. "Pituitary size in depression." Journal of Clinical Endocrinology and Metabolism 72, 2 (1999): 256-259.

70. S. Bhati and K. Richards. "A systematic review of the relationship between post-partum sleep disturbance and post-partum depression." Journal of Obstetric, Gynecologic, and Neonatal Nursing 44, 3 (2015): 350–57.

71. Michele Okun et al. "Sleep complaints in late pregnancy and the recurrence of post-partum depression." Behavioral Sleep Medicine 7, 2 (2009): 106–17.

72. John Csernansky et al. "Preclinical detection of alzheimer's disease: hippocampal shape and volume predict dementia onset in the elderly." NeuroImage 25, 3 (2005): 783–92.

73. David Bachman et al. "Incidence of dementia and probable alzheimer's disease in a general population the Framingham study." Neurology 43, 3 (1993): 515–515.

74. J. Douglas Bremner et al. "MRI and PET study of deficits in hippocampal structure and function in women with childhood sexual abuse and post-traumatic stress disorder." American Journal of Psychiatry 160, 5 (2003): 924–32.

75. Dieter Riemann et al. "Chronic insomnia and MRI-measured hippocampal volumes: a pilot study." Sleep 30, 8 (2007): 955–58.

76. Joost Janssen et al. "Hippocampal changes and white matter lesions in early-onset depression." Biological Psychiatry 56, 11 (2004): 825–31.

77. J. Douglas Bremner et al. "Hippocampal volume reduction in major depression." The American Journal of Psychiatry 157, 1 (2000): 115–18.

78. Anthony Jorm. "Is depression a risk factor for dementia or cognitive decline?" Gerontology 46, 4 (2000): 219–27.

79. Claire Burton et al. "The association of anxiety and depression with future dementia diagnosis: a case-control study in primary care." Fam Pract. 30,1 (2013): 25–30.

80. Theodore Kotchen et al. "Renin, norepinephrine, and epinephrine responses to graded exercise." Journal of Applied Physiology 31, 2 (1971): 178–84.

81. Kirsten Rennie et al. "Effects of moderate and vigorous physical activity on heart rate variability in a British study of civil servants." American Journal of Epidemiology 158, 2 (2003): 135–43.

82. Agneta Ståhle et al. "Aerobic group training improves exercise capacity and heart rate variability in elderly patients with a recent coronary event. a randomized controlled study." European Heart Journal 20, 22 (1999): 1638–46.

83. Wayne Levy et al. "Effect of endurance exercise training on heart rate variability at rest in healthy young and older men." The American Journal of Cardiology 82, 10 (1998): 1236–41.

84. Robinson Ramírez-Vélez et al. "Effect of moderate versus high-intensity interval exercise training on heart rate variability parameters in inactive Latin-American adults: a randomised clinical trial." Journal of Strength and Conditioning Research (2017).

85. Giselle Passos et al. "Effect of acute physical exercise on patients with chronic primary insomnia." Journal of Clinical Sleep Medicine 6, 3 (2010): 270–75.

86. Giselle Passos et al. "Effects of moderate aerobic exercise training on chronic primary insomnia." Sleep Medicine 12, 10 (2011): 1018–27.

87. Hooria Jazaieri et al. "A randomized trial of MBSR versus aerobic exercise for social anxiety disorder." Journal of Clinical Psychology 68, 7 (2012): 715–31.

88. Esther de Bruin et al. "A RCT comparing daily mindfulness meditations, biofeedback exercises, and daily physical exercise on attention control, executive functioning, mindful awareness, self-compassion, and worrying in stressed young adults." Mindfulness 7, 5 (2016): 1182–92.

89. D. McEntee & R. Halgin. Cognitive group therapy and aerobic exercise in the treatment of anxiety. Journal of College Student Psychotherapy 13,3 (1999): 37-55.

90. Andreas Ströhle et al. "The acute antipanic activity of aerobic exercise." The American Journal of Psychiatry 162, 12 (2005): 2376–78.

91. Andrea Dunn et al. "Exercise treatment for depression, efficacy and dose response" American Journal of Preventive Medicine 28, 1 (2005): 1–8.

92. Egil Martinsen et al. "Effects of aerobic exercise on depression: a controlled study." British Medical Journal (Clinical Research Ed.) 291, 6488 (1985): 109.

93. Chanudda Nabkasorn et al. "Effects of physical exercise on depression, neuroendocrine stress hormones and physiological fitness in adolescent females with depressive symptoms." European Journal of Public Health 16, 2 (2006): 179–84.

94. Alessandra Pilu et al. "Efficacy of physical activity in the adjunctive treatment of major depressive disorders: preliminary results." Clinical Practice and Epidemiology in Mental Health 3, 1 (2007): 3-8.

95. Michael Babyak et al., "Exercise treatment for major depression: maintenance of therapeutic benefit at 10 months." Psychosomatic Medicine 62, 5 (2000): 633.

96. Nalin Singh et al. "A randomized controlled trial of progressive resistance training in depressed elders." The Journals of Gerontology. Series A, Biological Sciences and Medical Sciences 52, 1 (1997): M27-35.

97. Nalin Singh et al. "A randomized controlled trial of high versus low intensity weight training versus general practitioner care for clinical depression in older adults." The Journals of Gerontology. Series A, Biological Sciences and Medical Sciences 60, 6 (2005): 768–76.

98. Elizabeth Doyne et al. "Running versus weight lifting in the treatment of depression." Journal of Consulting and Clinical Psychology 55, 5 (1987): 748.

99. Roma Robertson et al., "Walking for depression or depressive symptoms: a systematic review and meta- analysis." Mental Health and Physical Activity 5, 1 (2012): 66–75.

100. Ali Weinstein et al. "Heart rate variability as a predictor of negative mood symptoms induced by exercise withdrawal." Medicine and Science in Sports and Exercise 39, 4 (2007): 735–41.

101. Jeanne Molin et al. "The influence of climate on development of winter depression." Journal of Affective Disorders 37, 2 (1996): 151–55.

102. Katriina Kukkonen-Harjula et al. "Haemodynamic and hormonal responses to heat exposure in a Finnish sauna bath." European Journal of Applied Physiology and Occupational Physiology 58, 5 (1989): 543–50.

103. Krista Kauppinen et al. "Some endocrine responses to sauna, shower and ice water immersion." Arctic Medical Research 48, 3 (1989): 131–39.

104. Daniela Jezová et al. "Sex differences in endocrine response to hyper-thermia in sauna." Acta Physiologica Scandinavica 150, 3 (1994): 293–98.

105. So Kuwahata et al. "Improvement of autonomic nervous activity by Waon Therapy in patients with chronic heart failure." Journal of Cardiology 57, 1 (2011): 100–106.

106. Takashi Kihara et al. "Repeated sauna treatment improves vascular endothelial and cardiac function in patients with chronic heart failure." Journal of the American College of Cardiology 39, 5 (2002): 754–59.

107. Hiromitsu Miyamoto et al. "Safety and efficacy of repeated sauna bathing in patients with chronic systolic heart failure: a preliminary report." Journal of Cardiac Failure 11, 6 (2005): 432–36.

108. Shinya Hayasaka et al. "Effects of charcoal kiln saunas (Jjimjilbang) on psychological states." Complementary Therapies in Clinical Practice 14, 2 (2008): 143–48.

109. Akinori Masuda et al. "Repeated thermal therapy diminishes appetite loss and subjective complaints in mildly depressed patients." Psychosomatic Medicine 67, 4 (2005): 643.

110. Giresh Kanji et al. "Efficacy of regular sauna bathing for chronic tension-type headache: a randomized controlled study." Journal of Alternative and Complementary Medicine 21, 2 (2015): 103–9.

111. Ayesha A. Khanam et al. "Study of pulmonary and autonomic functions of asthma patients after yoga training." Indian Journal of Physiology and Pharmacology 40, 4 (1996): 318–24.

112. G. Pal et al. "Effect of short-term practice of breathing exercises on autonomic functions in normal human volunteers." The Indian Journal of Medical Research 120, 2 (2004): 115–21.

113. Shirley Telles et al. "Heart rate variability in chronic low back pain patients randomized to yoga or standard care." BMC Complementary and Alternative Medicine 16 (2016): 279.

114. M. Sawane and S. Gupta. "Resting heart rate variability after yogic training and swimming: a prospective randomized comparative trial." International Journal of Yoga 8, 2 (2015): 96.

115. N. Manjunath and S. Telles. "Influence of yoga and ayurveda on self-rated sleep in a geriatric population." The Indian Journal of Medical Research 121, 5 (2005): 683–90.

116. Michael Smith et al. "Comparative meta-analysis of pharmacotherapy and behavior therapy for persistent insomnia." American Journal of Psychiatry (2002): 5-11.

117. Gurminder Sahasi et al. "Effectiveness of yogic techniques in the management of anxiety." Journal of Personality and Clinical Studies 5, 1 (1989): 51–55.

118. M. Javnbakht et al. "Effects of yoga on depression and anxiety of women." Complementary Therapies in Clinical Practice 15, 2 (2009): 102–4.

119. S Parthasarathy et al. Effect of integrated yoga module on selected psychological variables among women with anxiety problem. West Indian Med J 63, 1 (2014): 78.

120. N. Janakiramaiah et al. "Therapeutic efficacy of Sudarshan Kriya Yoga (SKY) in dysthymic disorder." Nimhans Journal 16, 1 (1998): 21–28.

121. N. Janakiramaiah et al. "Antidepressant efficacy of Sudarshan Kriya Yoga (SKY) in melancholia: a randomized comparison with electroconvulsive therapy (ECT) and imipramine." Journal of Affective Disorders 57, 1–3 (2000): 255–59.

122. S. Khumar et al. "Effectiveness of Shavasana on depression among university students." Ind. J. Clin. Psychol. 20, 2 (1993): 82-87.

123. Lisa Butler et al. "Meditation with yoga, group therapy with hypnosis, and psychoeducation for long term depressed mood: a randomized pilot trial." Journal of Clinical Psychology 64, 7 (2008): 806–20.

124. Mahvash Shahidi et al. "Laughter yoga versus group exercise program in elderly depressed women: a randomized controlled trial." International Journal of Geriatric Psychiatry 26, 3 (2011): 322–27.

125. Prabhjot Nijjar et al. "Modulation of the autonomic nervous system assessed through heart rate variability by a mindfulness based stress reduction program." International Journal of Cardiology 177, 2 (2014): 557–59.

126. Jessica Del Pozo et al. "Biofeedback treatment increases heart rate variability in patients with known coronary artery disease." American Heart Journal 147, 3 (2004): 545.

127. Maura Paul-Labrador et al. "Effects of a randomized controlled trial of transcendental meditation on components of the metabolic syndrome in subjects with coronary heart disease." Archives of Internal Medicine 166, 11 (2006): 1218–24.

128. Jon Kabat-Zinn. "Mindfulness-based interventions in context: past, present, and future." Clinical Psychology: Science and Practice 10, 2 (2003): 144–56.

129. Ala'Aldin Al-Hussaini et al. "Vipassana meditation: A naturalistic, preliminary observation in Muscat." J Sci Res Med Sci. 3, 2 (2001): 87–92.

130. Tonya Jacobs et al. "Intensive meditation training, immune cell telomerase activity, and psychological mediators." Psychoneuroendocrinology 36, 5 (2011): 664–81.

131. R. Szekeres and E. Wertheim. "Evaluation of Vipassana meditation course effects on subjective stress, well-being, self-kindness and mindfulness in a community sample: post-course and 6-month outcomes." Stress and Health 31, 5 (2015): 373–81.

132. S. Wu and P. Lo. "Inward-attention meditation increases parasympathetic activity: a study based on heart rate variability." Biomedical Research 29, 5 (2008): 245–50.

133. Tetsuya Takahashi et al. "Changes in EEG and autonomic nervous activity during meditation and their association with personality traits." International Journal of Psychophysiology 55, 2 (2005): 199–207.

134. Auditya Sutarto et al. "Resonant breathing biofeedback training for stress reduction among manufacturing operators." International Journal of Occupational Safety and Ergonomics 18, 4 (2012): 549–561.

135. Chung-Kang Peng et al. "Heart rate dynamics during three forms of meditation." International Journal of Cardiology 95, 1 (2004): 19–27.

136. Crissa Guglietti et al. "Meditation-related increases in GABA B modulated cortical inhibition." Brain Stimulation 6 (2013) 397-402.

137. A Elias and A. Wilson. "Serum hormonal concentrations following transcendental meditation potential role of gamma aminobutyric acid." Medical Hypotheses 44 (1995): 287-291.

138. Cynthia Gross et al. "Mindfulness-based stress reduction vs. pharmacotherapy for primary chronic insomnia: a pilot randomized controlled clinical trial." Explore (N.Y.) 7, 2 (2011): 76–87.

139. Jason Ong et al. "A randomized controlled trial of mindfulness meditation for chronic insomnia." Sleep 37, 9 (2014): 1553–63.

140. J. Piet and E. Hougaard. "The effect of mindfulness- based cognitive therapy for prevention of relapse in recurrent major depressive disorder: a systematic review and meta-analysis." Clinical Psychology Review 31, 6 (2011): 1032–40.

141. Willem Kuyken et al. "Mindfulness-based cognitive therapy to prevent relapse in recurrent depression." Journal of Consulting and Clinical Psychology 76, 6 (2008): 966–78.

142. W. Lu and C. Kuo. "The effect of Tai Chi Chuan on the autonomic nervous modulation in older persons." Medicine and Science in Sports and Exercise 35, 12 (2003): 1972–76.

143. W. Lu and C. Kuo. "Effect of 3-month Tai Chi Chuan on heart rate variability, blood lipid and cytokine profiles in middle-aged and elderly individuals." International Journal of Gerontology 6, 4 (2012): 267–72.

144. Michael Irwin et al. "Improving sleep quality in older adults with moderate sleep complaints: a randomized controlled trial of Tai Chi Chuan." Sleep 31, 7 (2008): 1001–8.

145. Fuzhong Li et al. "Tai Chi and self rated quality of sleep and daytime sleepiness in older adults: a randomized controlled trial." Journal of the American Geriatrics Society 52, 6 (2004): 892–900.

146. M. Nguyen and A. Kruse. "A randomized controlled trial of Tai Chi for balance, sleep quality and cognitive performance in elderly Vietnamese." Clinical Interventions in Aging 7 (2012): 185–90.

147. Jen-Chen Tsai et al. "The beneficial effects of Tai Chi Chuan on blood pressure and lipid profile and anxiety status in a randomized controlled trial." Journal of Alternative and Complementary Medicine 9, 5 (2003): 747–54.

148. Kee-Lee Chou et al. "Effect of Tai Chi on depressive symptoms amongst Chinese older patients with depressive disorders: a randomized clinical trial." International Journal of Geriatric Psychiatry 19, 11 (2004): 1105–7.

149. Fang Wang et al. "The effects of Tai Chi on depression, anxiety, and psychological well-being: a systematic review and meta-analysis." International Journal of Behavioral Medicine 21, 4 (2014): 605–17.

150. F. López-Muñoz and C. Alamo. "Monoaminergic neurotransmission: the history of the discovery of antidepressants from 1950s until today." Current Pharmaceutical Design 15, 14 (2009): 1563–86.

151. Louis van Zyl et al. "Effects of antidepressant treatment on heart rate variability in major depression: a quantitative review." BioPsychoSocial Medicine 2 (2008): 12.

152. R. Noordam et al. "Antidepressants and heart-rate variability in older adults: a population-based study." Psychological Medicine 46, 6 (2016): 1239–47.

153. Johannes Terhardt et al. "Heart rate variability during antidepressant treatment with venlafaxine and mirtazapine." Clinical Neuropharmacology 36, 6 (2013):198–202.

154. Jordan Smoller et al. "Antidepressant use and risk of incident cardiovascular morbidity and mortality among postmenopausal women in the women's health initiative study." Archives of Internal Medicine 169, 22 (2009): 2128–39.

155. Wei-lun Huang et al. "The effects of antidepressants and quetiapine on heart rate variability." Pharmacopsychiatry 49, 5 (2016): 191–98.

156. Wing-FaiYeung. "Doxepin for insomnia: A systematic review of randomized placebo-controlled trials." Sleep Medicine Reviews 19 (2015): 75-83.

157. Nina Buscemi et al. "The efficacy and safety of drug treatments for chronic insomnia in adults: a meta-analysis of RCTs." Journal of General Internal Medicine 22, 9 (2007):1335.

158. Clifford Singer et al. "A multicenter, placebo-controlled trial of melatonin for sleep disturbance in Alzheimer's disease." Sleep 26, 7 (2003): 893.

159. Karl Rickels et al. "Long-term therapeutic use of benzodiazepines: i. effects of abrupt discontinuation." Archives of General Psychiatry 47, 10 (1990): 899–907.

160. Antoine Pélissolo et al. "Anxiety and depressive disorders in 4,425 long term benzodiazepine users in general practice." L'Encephale 33, 1 (2007): 32–38.

161. N. Koen and D. Stein. "Pharmacotherapy of Anxiety Disorders: A Critical Review." Dialogues in Clinical Neuroscience 13, 4 (2011): 423–37.

162. Murray Stein et al. "Efficacy of low and higher dose extended-release venlafaxine in generalized social anxiety disorder: a 6-month randomized controlled trial." Psychopharmacology 177, 3 (2005): 280–88.

163. Alan Gelenberg et al. "Efficacy of venlafaxine extended-release capsules in nondepressed outpatients with generalized anxiety disorder: a 6-month randomized controlled trial." JAMA 283, 23 (2000): 3082–88.

164. Serge Steenen et al. "Propranolol for the treatment of anxiety disorders: systematic review and meta-analysis." Journal of Psychopharmacology 30, 2 (2016): 128.

165. I. Kirsch and G. Sapirstein. "Listening to prozac but hearing placebo: a meta-analysis of antidepressant medication." Prevention & Treatment 1 (1998): 1-16.

166. BPAC. The role of medicines for the treatment of depression and anxiety in patients aged under 18 years. Best Practice Journal 74 (2016): 19-26.

167. Zindel Segal et al. "Antidepressant monotherapy versus sequential pharmacotherapy and mindfulness-based cognitive therapy, or placebo, for relapse prophylaxis in recurrent depression." Archives of General Psychiatry 67, 12 (2010): 1256–64.

168. Carlos Zarate et al. "A randomized trial of an N-Methyl-D-Aspartate antagonist in treatment-resistant major depression." Archives of General Psychiatry 63, 8 (2006): 856–64.

169. Nancy Diazgranados et al. "A randomized add-on trial of an N-Methyl-D-Aspartate antagonist in treatment- resistant bipolar depression." Archives of General Psychiatry 67, 8 (2010): 793–802.

170. Peter Nagele et al. "Nitrous oxide for treatment- resistant major depression: a proof-of-concept trial." Biological Psychiatry 78, 1 (2015): 10–18.

171. Bunmi Olatunji et al. "Efficacy of cognitive behavioral therapy for anxiety disorders: a review of meta- analytic findings." Psychiatric Clinics of North America, Cognitive Behavioral Therapy 33, 3 (2010): 557–77.

172. Irene Elkin et al. "National Institute of Mental Health treatment of depression collaborative research program: general effectiveness of treatments." Archives of General Psychiatry 46, 11 (1989): 971–82.

173. Sona Dimidjian et al. "Randomized trial of behavioural activation, cognitive therapy, and antidepressant medication in the acute treatment of adults with major depression." Journal of Consulting and Clinical Psychology 74, 4 (2006): 658–70.

NZ PAIN FOUNDATION

The NZ Pain Foundation was set up in 2013 to help people who suffer from mental and physical pain. Currently over 20 percent of the population suffer from common pain complaints such as headache, migraine, low back pain, neck pain, anxiety and depression with no answers. Most do not even know what is causing their symptoms. The NZ Pain Foundation hopes to foster research and education on self-treatments that are aimed at the cause of symptoms.

The NZ Pain Foundation was setup by Dr Giresh Kanji after completing a PhD, investigating how chronic pain spreads and amplifies with time. The Adrenaline Model of Headache Causation was formed which provides new information and directions for research for common conditions. He performed a clinical trial that showed regular attendance at a sauna was as effective as mainstream medication for people suffering from daily headache.

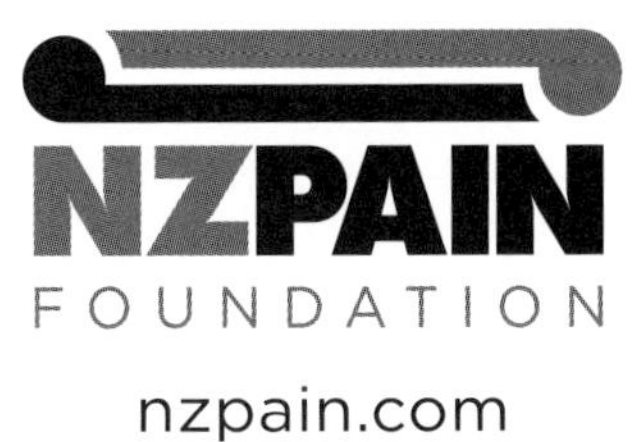

nzpain.com

Other books written by Dr Giresh Kanji

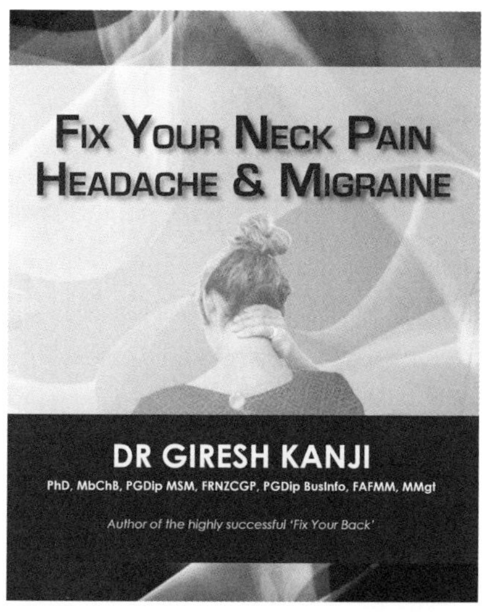

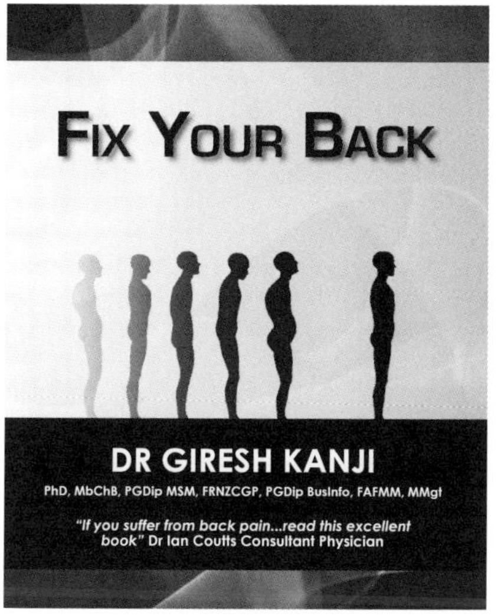